D1730800

Stability of Insulin

Studies on the physical and chemical stability of
insulin in pharmaceutical formulation

Jens Brange

Novo Research Institute
Novo Alle
DK-2880 Bagsværd
Denmark

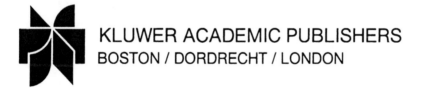

KLUWER ACADEMIC PUBLISHERS
BOSTON / DORDRECHT / LONDON

Denne afhandling er af Danmarks Farmaceutiske Højskole antaget til offentligt at forsvares for den farmaceutiske doktorgrad.

København, den 27. juni 1994

Birte Jensen

rektor

Forsvaret finder sted den 20. januar 1995 kl. 14.00 i Auditorium 4, Danmarks Farmaceutiske Højskole, Universitetsparken 2, København Ø.

This thesis has been accepted by the Royal Danish School of Pharmacy for public defence in fulfilment of the requirements for the degree Doctor of Pharmaciae (Dr. Pharm.).

Copenhagen, June 27, 1994

Birte Jensen

rector

The defence will take place on January 20th, 1995 at 2 p.m. in Auditorium 4, Danmarks Farmaceutiske Højskole, Universitetsparken 2, København Ø.

Distributors

for the United States and Canada: Kluwer Academic Publishers, PO Box 358, Accord Station, Hingham, MA 02018-0358, USA

for all other countries: Kluwer Academic Publishers Group, Distribution Center, PO Box 322, 3300 AH Dordrecht, The Netherlands

A catalogue record for this book is available from the British Library.

ISBN 0-7923-8977-8

List of the submitted publications

I. Brange J., Havelund S., Hansen P., Langkjaer L., Sørensen E., and Hildebrandt P., 1982, Formulation of physically stable neutral solutions for continuous infusion by delivery systems. In Hormone Drugs, Gueriguian JL, Bransome ED, Outschoorn AS, Eds, Rockville, MD, US Pharmacopoeial Convention, pp. 96-105.

II. Brange J., Havelund S., Hommel E., Sørensen E., and Kühl C., 1986, Neutral insulin solutions physically stabilized by addition of Zn^{2+}. Diabetic Med. 3:532-536.

III. Brange J., Langkjær L., Havelund S., and Vølund A., 1992, Chemical stability of insulin: 1. Hydrolytic degradation during storage of pharmaceutical preparations. Pharm. Res. 9:715-726.

IV. Brange J., Havelund S., and Hougaard P., 1992, Chemical stability of insulin: 2. Formation of higher molecular weight transformation products during storage of pharmaceutical insulin preparations. Pharm. Res. 9:727-734.

V. Brange J., and Langkjær L., 1992, Chemical stability of insulin: 3. Influence of excipients, formulation, and pH. Acta Pharm. Nord. 4:149-158.

VI. Brange J, 1992, Chemical stability of insulin: 4. Kinetics and mechanisms of the chemical transformation in pharmaceutical formulation. Acta Pharm. Nord. 4:209-222.

VII. Brange J., Hallund O., and Sørensen E., 1992, Chemical stability of insulin: 5. Isolation, characterization and identification of insulin transformation products. Acta Pharm. Nord. 4:223-232.

Preface and acknowledgements

The stability studies reported in the submitted 7 articles, as well as in other investigations discussed in this overview, were carried out at the Novo Research Institute and in the research laboratories of Novo Industri A/S. The work was initiated in 1969 at a time when insulin of unprecedented purity became available and made the studies possible.

I am grateful to Henrik Ege, Jørgen Schlichtkrull, Jan Leschly and Lise Heding for excellent working conditions over the many years these studies have been running.

Part of the investigations have been carried out in collaboration with colleagues at the institute, in Novo Industri A/S and at Hvidøre Hospital, and I am especially grateful to Ole Hallund who contributed with development of analytical methods, to Svend Havelund who did the same, and performed numerous HPLC analyses, to Lotte Langkjær and Philip E. Hansen for analytical assistance, to Aage Vølund and Philip Hougaard who made the statistical analyses, and to Else Sørensen who performed the biological investigations. I also want to thank Per Hildebrandt, Eva Hommel and Claus Kühl for performing and supervising the clinical studies.

I am especially grateful for the skillful technical assistance I received from Lene Grønlund Andersen, Lene Bramsen and Eva Bøg, but also Helle Arrøe, Jessie Frederiksen, Dorte Karkov, and Harriet Markussen, made important contributions.

I also want to express my gratitude to Rod E. Hubbard, Xiao Bing and Leif Nørskov-Lauritsen for their help and advice on molecular modelling, to Jørgen Elnegård for large scale separations, to Henning Jacobsen and Lars Thim for amino acid and sequence analyses, to Klavs Jørgensen, Per Balschmidt, and Francis C. Szoka for helpful discussions, and to Kathleen Larsen and Else Jørgensen for invaluable linguistic help.

Special thanks are due to Professor Guy Dodson for stimulating discussions and never failing enthusiasm and encouragement.

Finally, I want to express a sincere thank to my wife, Lotte Langkjær. Without her immense support, motivation and, not least, patience during the many years, the present work would never have been finished.

Contents

Introduction   6

I. Historical perspective   7
A. Introduction   7
B. Early observations relating to stability   7
C. Insulin purity   9

II. Scenario: structure of the insulin molecule   11
A. Primary structure   11
B. Secondary and tertiary structure   12
C. Quaternary structure (self-association)   12
D. Structure of insulin in pharmaceutical formulations   15

III. Studies on insulin stability   17
A. Introduction   17
B. Biological stability   17
C. Physical stability   18
    1. Introduction   18
    2. Insulin fibrillation   18
      a. Formation and properties of insulin fibrils   18
      b. Structure of fibrous insulin   19
      c. Prevention of insulin fibrillation   21
      d. Fibril formation *in vivo*   22
D. Chemical stability   23
    1. Introduction   23
    2. Formation of hydrolysis products   23
      a. Deamidation reactions   24
      b. Chain cleavage   26
    3. Di- and polymerization   28
      a. Amine reactions   28
      b. Disulfide interchange reactions   30
    4. Influence of pH and auxiliary substances   30
    5. Effect of temperature   30
    6. Kinetics and mechanisms   32
    7. Properties of transformation products   35
    8. Influence on the quality of pharmaceutical preparations   36
E. Structure–stability relationship   37

Summary and conclusion   37

Resumé og konklusion   42

References   46

Reproductions of submitted papers   60

Introduction

The medical importance, availability and relatively high purity of insulin has made this hormone one of the most extensively investigated biomolecules, studies with a profound impact on our understanding of proteins and their structure. Insulin, with the size of a peptide but having all the features of a globular protein, has been the subject of pioneering research into sequence[249,253], chemical synthesis[170,185,209] and three dimensional structure[4,15] of proteins.

Maintenance of the structural integrity of a therapeutical protein is essential for its efficacy in relation to physiological and pharmacological activity. The structural changes taking place during its handling, storage and use can be categorized into either involving physical or chemical alterations in the molecule. Physical instability refers to changes in conformation (secondary to quaternary structure), also called unfolding or 'denaturation'. Chemical instability involves covalent modification of the sequence (primary structure), i.e. bond formation or cleavage, leading to a new chemical entity. In practice, however, these two distinct routes of transformation of the structure have a mutual influence, as changes in conformation affect the susceptibility of the molecule for chemical attack and vice versa. The purpose of the present survey has been to review the literature dealing with stability of insulin in pharmaceutical formulation, and to summarize and collectively discuss the author's own work in this field which has previously been published in a number of papers. These investigations were initiated at a time when the author was involved in the development of chromatographic purification of insulin which, during the years 1968–1975, led to a substantial and important improvement in insulin purity (monocomponent or MC-insulin[261]). This advancement was essential for the evaluation of the chemical stability of insulin, in particular.

I. Historical perspective

A. INTRODUCTION

The term 'Insulin' was introduced before 'the internal secretion of the pancreas' was an established fact, and the stability of the hormone was an important issue long before insulin was finally successfully isolated by Banting and coworkers in 1921. Based upon the gdemonstrated relationship between the pancreas and diabetes mellitus in 1890[212], numerous attempts were made in the following many years to demonstrate that extracts of the pancreas were able to alleviate or remove the symptoms of diabetes. But the search for insulin during this thirty-year period was unsuccessful as the results obtained were either negative or not favorable enough to justify further experimentation. The endeavors probably failed because the active principle was degraded by the enzymes present in the pancreatic extracts or because the majority of these early attempts used oral administration of the extracts. In both cases the result was destruction of the insulin activity by digestive enzymes.

It is interesting to note that some of these workers made predictions about the stability of insulin. Thus in 1911 Drennan[94] observed that intravenous injection of defibrinated blood from a normal dog into a pancreatectomized dog lost its effect on lowering the content of sugar in the urine if the defibrinated blood had been stored for a few hours before injection, and he concluded: "The internal secretion of the normal pancreas appears to be a relatively unstable body, a fact which may make its extraction from the gland difficult, and may account for some of the failures to secure active extracts from the pancreas." Scott[269] was of the opinion that the active principle was so unstable that it ceased to exist as soon as it was removed from the cells, and in 1912 Knowlton and Starling[177] stated: "Reasoning from the behavior of such substances as the class of hormones, such as secretin and adrenaline, we might guess that the pancreatic hormone would be a body, diffusible, soluble in water, unstable in alkaline solution, but more stable in slightly acid solution and not destroyed at the temperature of boiling water."

B. EARLY OBSERVATIONS RELATING TO STABILITY

Already the original inventors noted that the potency of their extracts was destroyed by boiling and by pancreatic juice[17-19], but, on the other hand, was not affected by the presence of tricresol[18]. It was early confirmed by several investigators that the physiological activity of insulin was destroyed by proteolytic enzymes, such as pepsin[95,102, 109,139,328,333] and trypsin [95,103,139,266,277,333].

During the decade following the first successful extraction of insulin most of the chemical and physical experiments on insulin were attempts to obtain the active principle in as pure form as possible, and to determine some of its general chemical characteristics in an endeavor to elucidate its chemical nature and the composition of the active principle. The problem of establishing a relationship between biological activity and the presence of certain groups in the molecule was approached by blocking the active group or groups by chemical derivation, or by splitting off supposedly active groups. In undertaking such experiments useful information about the stability of the active principle was also obtained. From these early investigations it was evident that insulin is unstable towards alkali, but is relatively stable in acid. Thus Murlin et al.[218] found that boiling in acid medium for five minutes did not destroy the active principle, whereas slow inactivation occurred when the heating was extended to 1–2 hours[95] or if the acid solution was autoclaved[80]. Moderate degrees of alkalinity did not affect the strength of insulin during a period of 6 minutes at room temperature[28]. Dudley[95] observed complete destruction of the active principle after 1.5 h at 37°C when extracts were incubated in 0.1 N NaOH, whereas some activity was retained after the same treatment in 0.1 N sodium carbonate. Attempts to reactivate alkali-treated insulin were generally unsuccessful[158,276], although partial recovery was sometimes observed after treatment in ammonium hydroxide[277,334]. Liberation of ammonia was observed during treatment with acid as well as alkali[58,118,156,159]. However, it was already at that time realized that the inactivation in alkali was associated with alterations in the sulfur of the hormone[2,37,120], and the destructive action of sulphydryl compounds on the physiological activity was well established[312,332].

At the time when crystalline and, therefore, relatively pure insulin preparations were becoming available, it was found that heating insulin in acid provoked insulin to precipitate in an inactive form[32,34,76,90,124,182,310]. The phenomenon was termed heat denaturation or coagulation, but it was shown later that heat precipitation and insulin fibrillation are directly related[319]. The precipitate was shown to be insoluble in acid but to resume its original solubility and activity in dilute alkali[34,90,310], wherefore the phenomenon was believed by some investigators to be due to a reversible chemical process[68,76,124]. The tendency to heat inactivation of the acid insulin solutions used for therapy at that time varied quite unpredictably, and therefore every lot had to be tested and meet certain requirements. The test was performed by exposing the acid solution to a temperature of 52°C for 10 days followed by bioassay, and it was found that insulin freed from metal ions lost more than 50% of its biological activity[251]. On the other hand, if zinc ions or certain other metal ions were added deterioration seemed to proceed at a slower rate[251,252]. It was also found that inactivation varied with the area of the solution exposed to air[252]. However, these results could not be confirmed in later experiments[192].

The storage stability of the acid insulin solutions used for therapy has apparently not been studied systematically during the first years of the insulin era, as no reports have been found in the literature. Only anecdotical mention of the shelf life has appeared. Thus Banting and Best[17] note that extract kept in cold storage retains its potency for at least seven days, and Macleod[200] states: "Order

Table 1   Advancement of the purity of insulin

Period	Insulin	Content of impurities (%)			Biological potency (IU/mg)
		HMWP[a]	CID[b] + Proinsulin[c]	Desamido-insulin	
1922–30	amorphous	> 30	?	> 15	
	1.Intern. Stand. (1923)	?	?	?	8
1930–50	once crystallized	5–10	5–8	5–15	
	2.Intern.Stand. (1935)	?	?	?	22
1950–70	recrystallized	0.2–2.5	3–6	5–15	
	4.Intern.Stand. (1958)	0.3	4	15	25.4
1970–75	once chromatographed	0.3–0.5	1–2	1–15	
1975–	rechromatographed	< 0.1	CID: < 0.2 Proinsulin: < 1 ppm	< 1	
	1. Intern. Stand. of human insulin (1987)	< 0.1	CID: 0.2 Proinsulin: < 1 ppm	< 1	28.1

[a] Higher-molecular-weight-products including pancreatic proteins and insulin derivatives
[b] Covalent insulin dimers; [c] Proinsulin + proinsulin derivatives

insulin sufficient for one month. It will not deteriorate." (and added the warning: "allow plenty of time for delay in mails"!). Later Choay[81], based on convulsion assay in a few rabbits, concluded that no appreciable change in activity of acid preparations could be observed after storage at room temperature for 18 months.

C. INSULIN PURITY

The yields and the purity of the first extracts were low[161] (Table 1), and data concerning the properties of these extremely heterogenous preparations of the hormone were obviously inexact until Abel in 1926[1] succeeded in crystallizing insulin and, thereby, improving its purity substantially. During the next four decades only minor advancement in the purity and, hence, the biological potency of the hormone took place. These improvements were mainly achieved by introduction of Zn^{2+}-crystallization[268] and recrystallization methods, the latter based on the observation that insulin recrystallized several times was better tolerated by patients suffering from allergic reactions[166]. Until the late 1960's recrystallized insulin was considered to be an essentially pure substance, but the introduction of new analytical methods made it possible to detect the presence of significant amounts of protein impurities by disc electrophoresis[215] and gel filtration[288,289]. The purity of recrystallized insulin, as revealed by these methods, was only 80–90%[45] (Table 1) rendering exact assessment of chemical stability extremely difficult. Therefore, a prerequisite for the present studies, as regards the chemical stability, has been the introduction of monocomponent (MC) insulins[261] which are, by chromatographic methods, purified to the extent that impurities are virtually undetectable by the above mentioned methods. The introduction of chromatographical purification reduced the content of impurities by at least one order of magnitude to less than 0.5%. The progress in biological potency (Table 1) is also substantial, but does not fully reflect the progress in chemical purity, which is due to the fact that several of the impurities removed by the chromatographical processes possess some or even full biological activity[45,53].

II. Scenario: structure of the insulin molecule

A. PRIMARY STRUCTURE

The human insulin molecule contains 51 amino acid residues in two polypeptide chains (A and B) linked by 2 disulfide bonds as illustrated in Figure 1. The A-chain consists of 21 residues with an additional disulfide loop between A6 and A11, whereas the longer B-chain holds 30 residues. Primary structures are now known for insulins from more than 50 animal species. Insulins from the hystricomorph rodent family show the highest number of amino acid

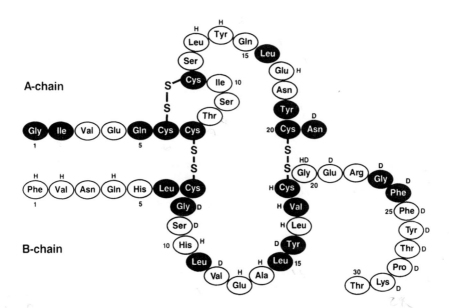

Figure 1. The primary structure of human insulin. The black residues designate the amino acids which are invariant among species of insulin. The superscripts indicate the residues involved in association of the molecule: D = dimer formation; H = hexamer formation. Porcine insulin only differs in position B30 (Ala instead of Thr). Bovine insulin has the same substitution and contains, in addition, Ala in position A8 and valine in position A10. (Adapted from ref. 54 with permission).

substitutions; guinea pig insulin, for example, contains 18 residues different from the respective positions in human insulin. Of the other insulins used for pharmaceutical preparations, porcine and bovine insulins contain alanine in position B30 and bovine insulin contains, in addition, alanine in A8 and valine in position A10.

The invariant residues (10 in each chain, see Figure 1) are typically the residues responsible for the structural integrity of the molecule and which help to define the folding of the molecule, e.g. the cystine residues, the nonpolar residues constituting the hydrophobic core, important for maintaining the molecule's structure, and other residues interacting in the folding of the molecule into its three- dimensional structure.

B. SECONDARY AND TERTIARY STRUCTURE

Despite variations in primary structure the folding and packing of the two chains into their three-dimensional conformation are essentially the same in all insulins. The A-chain forms two nearly antiparallel α helices, A2 to A8 and A13 to A20. The B-chain normally forms a single α-helix from B9 to B19 followed by a turn and a β-strand from B21 to B30. The arrangement of the chains buries the cystine A6–A11 and the aliphatic side chains of residues A2, A16, B11 and B15 which provide the molecule with a hydrophobic interior. Numerous non-covalent interactions between the amino acid residues of the two chains stabilize the tertiary structure. The surface of the insulin monomer is covered by both polar and nonpolar residues. Whereas the A-chain and the B9–B19 helix form a stable structural unit, the B25–B30 and the B1–B8 segments are variable in conformation. This three dimensional structure was established by X-ray analysis of Zn insulin crystals[4,15,35], but there is strong evidence that essentially the same structure applies to the circulating monomer[30,141] which binds to the insulin receptor. Also certain structural transformations induced by specific additives in threshold concentrations seem to be equivalent in solution and crystals[242]. Later studies by NMR spectroscopy have revealed a minor but distinct difference between the peripheral conformation of the free monomer and that of insulin in aggregated forms[248].

Recently it has been discovered that the presence of ∼1% phenol promotes formation of an additional helical segment from B1 to B8[87,284,335]. This structural transformation, involving movement of more than 25 Å at residue B1, only occurs when insulin is associated into hexamers[87]. Figure 2 shows the structure of the insulin monomer with and without this extra α-helix.

C. QUATERNARY STRUCTURE (SELF-ASSOCIATION)

Insulin exists as a monomer only at low concentration ($< 0.1 \mu M \sim 0.6 \mu g/ml$). It dimerizes at higher concentrations relevant for pharmaceutical formulation, and in the pH range 4–8, in the presence of zinc ions, three dimers assemble at concentrations above 0.01 mM further into a hexamer (Figure 3). At concentrations $\geq 2mM$ the hexamer is formed at neutral pH without assistance of zinc ions[136].

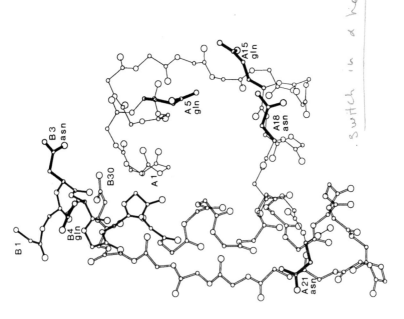

switch in α helix

Figure 2. Tertiary structures of the insulin molecule. The panels show the peptide backbone atoms of the A- and B-chains and their arrangements in the three-dimensional packing of the molecule. The A-chain is drawn with thin bonds. The B-chain from B1 to B8 is drawn with thick lines and the rest of the B-chain with open lines. Only the side chains of the six potentially labile amide residues are shown (thick lines). Left: The 'normal' most common structure with extended B-chain N-terminal. Right: The structure with a switch into α-helix of residues B1 to B8 promoted by phenol or phenol derivatives.

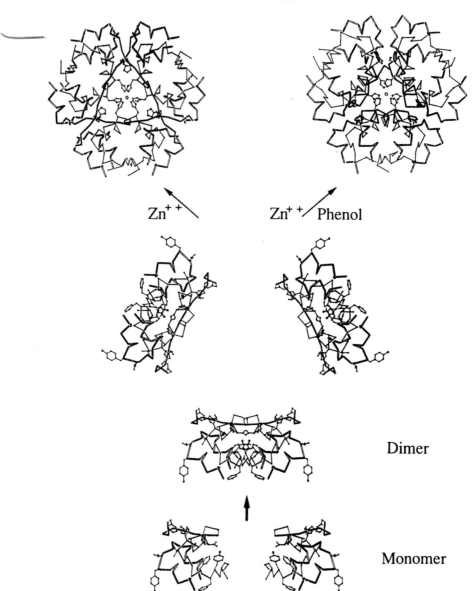

Figure 3. The self-assembly of insulin from the monomer to the dimer, and of three dimers into a hexamer in the presence of zinc ions. When, in addition, phenol (or phenol derivatives like *m*-cresol) is present the gathering of the three dimers is accompanied by a conformational transformation of B1 to B8 from an extended chain into an α-helix. Only the α-carbon atoms of the main chains are indicated. The A-chains are drawn with open bonds, the B-chain with thinner full bonds, and B1–B8 with thick bonds. The atoms in the side chains interacting in the dimer- and hexamer formation (see Figure 1) are drawn with thin bonds (adapted from ref. 54 with permission).

The two insulin molecules in the dimer are held together by predominantly nonpolar forces, reinforced by four hydrogen bonds (between B24 and B26 main chain atoms), in an antiparallel β-sheet structure between the two C-terminal strands of the B chain. This arrangement pulls the two insulin molecules together compactly and the dimer is stable in aqueous solutions between pH 2–8.

The packing of three dimers around two zinc ions is associated with the burial of the remaining nonpolar surface (A13–14, B1–2, B14 and B17–18), but the interactions between dimers in the hexamer are considerably looser than those between the monomers in the dimer. The hexamer, in which the A-chain constitutes a large proportion of the mostly polar surface, forms an almost spheric structure with a diameter of 50 Å and a height of about 35 Å. The zinc ions are situated in the polar channel in the center of the hexamer coordinated to B10 histidines. The above mentioned structural transition induced by phenol requires the presence of zinc ions and thus is a property of the hexamer. The phenol molecules bind in nonpolar cavities in the interface between dimers created by packing of A-chain residues from one dimer and the B1–B8 helical segment from the adjacent dimer. Six phenol molecules bind specifically to the hexamer, one to each monomer. The phenolic hydroxyl group is hydrogen bonded to a carbonyl oxygen of an A-chain Cys residue, whereas its hydrophobic end is in close proximity to the B3 Asn side chain of each monomer[87,284].

D. STRUCTURE OF INSULIN IN PHARMACEUTICAL FORMULATIONS

Today almost all insulin formulations are either neutral solutions or neutral suspensions of zinc insulin containing 40, 80 or 100 IU/ml (U-100 ~ 0.6 mM ≈ 4mg/ml). Consequently, these pharmaceutical preparations all share the hexamer of insulin as the common structural unit.

The formulation of rapid-acting insulin preparations (Regular insulin) varies with respect to the excipients added to the neutral solution of hexameric insulin. The original neutral solution[260] contains NaCl and methylparaben (Regular I), whereas a later version is formulated with glycerol and phenol or m-cresol (Regular II). In the latter formulation the phenol content most likely creates the aforementioned α-helix, whereas the propensity of methylparaben to induce the same change is very much reduced[335].

The potential of insulin to crystallize in a variety of forms, a reflection of the molecule's diverse association patterns and ligand binding properties, has been utilized in the formulations with retarded onset of action[45]. Although crystals of the insulin monomer, dimer and hexamer have all been obtained[87] the common unit in the pharmaceutically relevant crystals is the hexamer.

When a neutral solution of hexameric zinc insulin, in the presence of phenol (or m-cresol), is mixed with protamine, an arginine rich and therefore strongly basic polypeptide (M.W. approx. 4,300 D) isolated from salmon sperm, a precipitate is formed which converts to orthorhombic crystals with a strong tetragonal appearance[14,181]. These crystals contain approximately 0.9 molecules of protamine and 2 zinc atoms per insulin hexamer. The protamine is rather loosely bound in the crystal but mediates interactions between dimers in the hexamer, where it penetrates the polar central channel. In the interstices between hexamers it is also involved in hexamer–hexamer contacts[16,279]. Six *m*-cresol molecules occupy cavities in the hexamer created by A-chain residues from one dimer and the B1–B8 helical structure from the adjacent dimer[16]. The pharmaceutical preparation based on this principle is known as NPH (Neutral Protamine Hagedorn) or Isophane insulin and has an intermediate release profile after subcutaneous injection.

Gradation of the prolongation of the release of insulin was accomplished with the Lente insulin principle[134], also named Insulin Zinc Suspensions (IZS). It is based on the discovery that a protracted effect, depending on the physical state of the insulin, could be obtained by addition of small amounts of extra zinc ions to hexameric 2 zinc insulin in neutral medium. Amorphously precipitated zinc insulin complex (Semilente or IZS, amorphous) shows a slight retardation, whereas rhombohedral insulin crystals show a very prolonged action profile when additional zinc ions are added (Ultralente or IZS, crystalline). An intermediate action profile was obtained with a 3:7 mixture of amorphous and crystalline insulin particles (Lente or IZS, mixed).

III. Studies on insulin stability

A. INTRODUCTION

Insulin has been in therapeutic use for more than 70 years, but in the past its stability in pharmaceutical formulation has especially been systematically studied in terms of biological potency[233,291,293] but without investigations of the chemistry giving rise to the changes observed. Whereas the physical stability of insulin solutions under a variety of conditions has been extensively investigated throughout the years, primarily in connection with their more recent use in infusion pumps (see section III C 2), very little information has appeared in the literature on the chemical transformation of insulin during storage of insulin preparations. The few investigations in the past have all dealt with its hydrolysis in acid medium into insulin desamido products[27,280,296].

B. BIOLOGICAL STABILITY

Estimation of the biological potency of insulin was for many years the only way to evaluate the influence of different storage conditions on the stability of the hormone. Whereas the first investigations, dealing with acid solutions, were carried out only for short periods at elevated temperatures[182,193,251,252], more systematic studies were later carried out at temperatures encountered under ordinary storage conditions for the expected shelf life of the preparations[233,258,291,293]. Studying a whole range of acid and neutral insulin formulations including rapid-, intermediate- and long-acting preparations during storage at a variety of temperatures, Pingel and Vølund[233] found that all formulations exhibited a remarkably high stability of biological potency as, e.g., all preparations retained virtually full biological potency after five years of storage at 4°C. They also confirmed earlier observations that loss of biological potency follows a first order reaction[182,258,293] and that neutral insulin solutions are more stable than acid solutions[293]. The rate of biological inactivation was found to increase four- to fifteenfold by a temperature increase of 10°C, and the activation energy, E_a, was calculated to range from 117 to 179 kJ/mol[233].

C. PHYSICAL STABILITY

1. Introduction

Like other globular proteins, insulin tends to adopt and maintain a three-dimensional structure in which its hydrophobic surfaces are buried by folding or assembly of individual molecules. However, changes of the native conformation or of its 'normal' pattern of assembly can be provoked by a variety of factors. The most frequent events encountered in handling or use of insulin are increase in solution viscosity, precipitation from solutions, changes in physical appearance of suspensions and loss of insulin due to adsorption to surfaces. These phenomena have recently been reviewed[45,54] and only the propensity of insulin, especially under the influence of heat, to undergo conformational changes resulting in linear aggregation (fibrillation) and formation of a viscous gel or insoluble precipitates will be discussed in the following.

2. Insulin fibrillation

a. Formation and properties of insulin fibrils

The first systematic study of the heat precipitation of insulin was published by Krogh and Hemmingsen[182], who found the rate of inactivation at pH 3 to be proportional to the insulin concentration and to closely follow the law of Arrhenius in the temperature interval 50–117°C. Subsequent studies showed the rate of reaction in acid to be slowest between pH 2.6 and 3.3[124], and to be dependent of the type of acid (H_2SO_4 > HCl > H_3PO_4 >> HAc)[124,313].

Waugh[188,317] was the first to realize that formation of insulin fibers precedes precipitation and that the heat treatment does not radically alter the globular nature of the insulin molecule. He later showed that heat precipitation involves three reactions: formation of active centers (nucleation), elongation of these centers to fibrils (growth), and floccule formation (precipitation)[319,320,324]. The nucleation reaction, which is the slowest process, requires the nearly simultaneous interaction of 3–4 insulin molecules[326]. Essentially undistorted insulin is involved in these interactions which mainly are between non-polar side chains (hydrophobic interactions)[318,319,324]. The subunits of these interactions have been suggested to be either the dimer or the monomer of insulin[63,324]. Whereas nucleation seems to require temperature above normal, the growth into fibrils can proceed at ambient or even lower temperatures. Dependent on the conditions, in particular the ion strength, the growth leads to long fibers resulting in a thixotropic gel or to shorter fibers with a tendency to arrange radially to spherolites with precipitation as the consequence[324,326]. The growth of fibrils has been found to be a function of the surface area of the fibril population and the concentration of insulin in solution[325], and thus is a highly cooperative process able to quantitatively remove the insulin from solution in the fibrous form. Fibril formation has therefore been suggested as an *in vitro* assay for insulin[132,323], but such an assay is only applicable with preparations of substantially pure insulin as recoveries may be erratic in the presence of foreign proteins[117,194]. Fibril formation followed by regeneration in cold alkali has also been suggested as a means to purify insulin[230].

An increase in ionic strength increases the rate of nucleation as well as growth, whereas high concentrations of organic acids, urea and phenol suppress the nucleation reaction while allowing the growth reaction to proceed[324]. Whereas the rate of insulin fibrillation in acid, as would be expected, increases with insulin concentration[326], neutral solutions of hexameric insulin exhibit a quite anomalous aggregation behavior in being more prone to fibrillation at reduced concentration of insulin[41,86,282]. In sharp contrast, if zinc-free insulin in neutral solution is monomerized by introduction of 60% ethanol, the extent and rate of aggregation is proportional to insulin concentration[46]. Therefore, formation of fibril nuclei probably proceeds via monomerization of oligomeric insulin. This is supported by the fact that hydrophobic surfaces like air–water or plastic–water interfaces increase the tendency to fibrillation[38,86,108,198,282,283,302], probably via interaction with and subsequent exposure of the insulin monomer's hydrophobic interfaces normally buried in the dimer or hexamer[302]. The promoting effect of organic solvents, which weaken the hydrophobic interactions in native insulin and dissociate the insulin assemblies, on the formation of insulin fibrils can probably be ascribed to the same phenomenon.

Insulin fibrils are insoluble in most aqueous media, including diluted mineral acids. They can be dissolved and regenerated (renatured) into essentially fully biologically active insulin in alkaline medium at pH>11, followed by neutralization[160,313,322], in 20% HCl[311], in at least 10% phenol[326,192] or by using strong, organic acids[324]. In contrast, insulin fibrils are not dissolved in 7M urea from pH 2–8[229] or in 5M guanidine HCl, 50% acetonitrile, and non-ionic and anionic detergents[228]. Waugh[322] found the optimal conditions for regeneration in alkali to be treatment in 0.03M NaOH at 0°C for 45 minutes, and that NaCl inhibits reversion.

Human, porcine and bovine insulins vary in their tendency to form insulin fibrils, bovine insulin being more prone to fibrillation than the other two species of insulin. Apparently the A8 residue (Ala in bovine and Thr in porcine and human insulin), which is on the surface of the hexamer, plays a role in directing the interactions of insulin with hydrophobic surfaces, the first steps in the fibrillation process. The presence of certain types of inert protein was early shown to retard the rate of fibril formation although no conclusive evidence of the influence of purity could be obtained[124]. Later, following the introduction of monocomponent insulin in the 70's[261], a strong reverse relationship between the tendency to fibrillation and the content of insulin related impurities was demonstrated, and it was shown that this effect was not a result of the purification processes as such. If the impurities were reintroduced into monocomponent insulin the former propensity to less fibrillation could be re-established. It was also shown that higher molecular contaminants such as covalent dimer, proinsulin, etc. were most effective in counteracting fibrillation[38].

b. Structure of fibrous insulin

In the electron microscope insulin fibrils are seen as long fibers with the smallest diameters ranging from 3 to 15 nm[45,106,125,184,228,319,326] and lengths up to several microns[106,125]. Sometimes the individual fibrils are seen as bundles of two to five fibers twisted together at 120–160 nm intervals into filaments with a gross diameter of 10–20 nm[106,125,184].

Fibrous insulin has been studied by various techniques including spectroscopic and diffraction techniques. Using infra-red technique insulin fibrils were shown to consist of extended β-chains lying perpendicular to the fibril axis, with a layer structure involving inter-chain hydrogen bonds[8]. In contrast, from an X-ray diffraction investigation it was suggested that insulin enters the fibril structure with, at most, slight distortion, and without the large changes accompanying transformation to the β-form. It was also suggested that the polypeptide chains in insulin fibrils retain their normal folded condition, with axes predominantly parallel to the fibril axis[178]. Raman spectra of insulin fibrils[339] and studies of the binding of Congo Red to fibrillar insulin[306] gave evidence of an antiparallel β-structure, whereas infrared spectroscopy[125] and X-ray diffraction data[63] pointed to the parallel pleated-sheet type. The latter investigators also suggested that the fibrils had a uniform cross section with dimensions of about 30 by 50 Å.

Using dynamic light scattering technique it has recently been found that insulin fibrils are of narrow size distribution with a mean diameter of 200 nm[86]. Whereas the initial steps in association of insulin monomers into fibril nuclei probably are common for any insulin fibril formation, the further growth (aggregation) into macroscopic fibrils depends on the experimental conditions[45,147,256]. Based on computer simulations of insulin aggregation, a mechanism for fibrillation has recently been proposed[282,283] in which partially unfolded insulin monomers associate and form intermediate assemblies. When such intermediate fibril nuclei have reached a critical size (170 nm in diameter corresponding to approx. 100 insulin molecules) they have sufficient surface area for stability and for interactions with native insulin. The lag phase, often observed in insulin fibrillation experiments, was explained by the slow formation of stable intermediates as no significant aggregation was noticed until a population of nucleating species was established.

The specific amino acid residues involved in the interactions between units in fibrillar insulin have yet to be identified. Fibrillation experiments on different insulin derivatives have shown that fibril formation is not dependent on the presence of carboxyl groups[216,324], whereas a marked decrease in the tendency to fibrillation is observed when the amino groups are acetylated[159,324]. Studies on chemical reactivity of functional groups have revealed that about half of the imidazolyl[229,235] and half of the tyrosyl groups[229] have reduced reactivity in fibrillar as compared to native insulin. Subsequent iodination studies indicated the masked tyrosyl groups in fibrillar insulin to be mainly located in the A-chain[287]. More recent studies have shown that the B-chain C-terminal residues, essential for insulin dimer association, are not required for the interactions in insulin fibrils. On the contrary, if five or eight residues are removed from the C-terminal the propensity to fibril formation increases with increasing truncation. If, on the other hand, the B-chain C-terminal loses its flexibility partly (i.e. proinsulin) or wholly (i.e. miniproinsulin) by linking the terminal to the nearby A-chain N-terminal, the fibrillation process proceeds more slowly or not at all, respectively. These results strongly suggest that fibril nucleation requires exposure of the hydrophobic amino acid residues A2 Ile, B11 Leu and B15 Leu, normally buried in the insulin monomer, to the surface of the insulin molecule by displacement of the B-chain C-terminal from its normal position[46].

c. Prevention of insulin fibrillation

During the first 60 years of insulin therapy fibrillation-related stability problems during normal handling, storage or use of insulin preparations were rarely encountered, presumably, as no mention in the literature has been found. In the late 1970's the endeavors to obtain normoglycemia in diabetes treatment resulted in the introduction of continuous insulin infusion devices (insulin pumps) which were either worn externally[74,148,231,298] or implanted[60,61,66,112,149,257]. Use of insulin solutions in such systems involved the exposure of insulin to a combination of increased temperatures for extended periods of time, hydrophobic surfaces and, because of the movement of the devices, to shear forces. Together, these factors substantially increased the propensity of the insulin to form precipitates due to fibril formation. It soon became evident that commercial insulin formulations were not sufficiently stable for long-term use in infusion pumps[55,61,148,153,197]. Precipitation problems became of major concern and a comprehensive search for more stable formulations was started.

Numerous ways of stabilizing insulin solutions for use in delivery systems against fibrillation were investigated in the following years. These include the addition of autologous serum[5] or whole blood[138], use of organic media such as glycerol[33,60], introduction of organic[40,56,78,126,129,137,197,198,237,254,301,302] or inorganic additives[38,39,40,44,98,153,208,239], and derivatization of insulin[6,197,234,301]. Most of these methods are either impractical, inconvenient, or unsafe, in the sense that the additives used are unphysiological or have a deteriorating effect on the chemical and biological stability of the insulin. Thus addition of glycerol[60] as well as certain polysaccharides[40] significantly increases the physical stability of neutral insulin solutions, but, unfortunately, the physical stabilization is accompanied by an unacceptable decrease in the chemical and biological stability of the preparations[38-40]. It is now well recognized that polyols are able to stabilize the native structure of globular proteins[10,13,122,123,191]. However, in relation to prevention of insulin fibrillation, the stabilizing effect of polyols seems to be correlated with the capacity of these products to react chemically with the insulin amino groups. Hence aldoses are more effective than ketoses[40] and the deteriorating effect of glycerol is related to its content of aldehyde impurities[45]. Consequently, the inhibitory effect of these additives on insulin fibrillation is probably due, at least partly, to the preventive effect protein impurities have, as mentioned earlier, on the fibrillation process[38]. Recently it has been demonstrated that an increase of the viscosity of insulin solutions by addition of 15% (W/W) of polygeline counteracts the promoting effect of shear forces on insulin fibrillation[129]. Elevated viscosity probably has an impact on the rate of conformational changes[9] necessary for formation of insulin fibrils.

Addition of calcium and zinc ions, which probably also play an important role for the storage stability of insulin in the β cells of the pancreas[146], significantly improves the physical stability of neutral insulin solutions, especially at higher concentrations of insulin[38,44]. These metal ions probably exert their fibrillation-inhibitory effect by neutralizing negative charges in the center of the insulin

Table 2   Physical stabilization of neutral insulin solutions

Zinc ions / Hexamer	DOPC concentration (µg/ml)	Days to precipitation in shaking test (37°C)
0	0	< 1
2.2		1
2.9		1.5
3.9		20
2.2	30	18
2.9		32
3.9		40
4.6		>100

Stabilization against insulin fibrillation by addition of additional zinc ions and of the semisynthetic lecithin, dioctanoylphosphatidylcholine (DOPC). (Data from ref. 45 and 54)

hexamer[100,225,295] whereby the hexameric assembly is stabilized, without compromising the chemical stability[41,44]. A marked fibrillation-inhibitory effect is obtained by low concentrations of lecithins[137] or of a synthetic detergent[126,128]. The positive influence of detergent additives is based on their ability to inhibit adsorption of insulin onto hydrophobic surfaces which, subsequently, may lead to exposure of insulin's hydrophobic surfaces and structural rearrangement[302]. Most effective stabilization is seen when this method is combined with elevation of the viscosity of the solution[129] or with metal ion stabilization[54] (Table 2).

The influence of materials used in delivery systems on the tendency of insulin to fibrillate has been studied by several groups[38,78,108,129,271], and also the chemical stability of insulin in delivery systems environment or in contact with materials used in such systems has been reported[33,127,128,129,211,271]. These investigations have revealed that not only does the stability vary with the type and origin of the material in a very complex manner, but it is also dependent on the method by which the material has been sterilized[211].

d. Fibril formation in vivo

The term 'amyloid' is used to designate a pathologic proteinaceous substance deposited in tissue of patients suffering from a variety of inflammatory or degenerative clinical conditions. The most characteristic ultrastructural feature of amyloid deposits is accumulation of linear fibrils composed of a protein with chains arranged in a β-pleated sheet conformation[83,299]. This morphological similarity with insulin fibrils formed in vitro led to the suspicion that insulin is the source of pancreatic amyloid fibrils and may provide the subunits of such deposits[125,171]. Pancreatic islet amyloidosis has been detected in association with normal aging, type II diabetes or β-cell adenomas[97,163,330], and evidence for its relationship with insulin or insulin related proteins has been substantiated in a number of studies[171,222,264,329-331].

Local amyloidosis caused iatrogenically during insulin therapy, and dependent on the presence of insulin, has been demonstrated after continuous subcutaneous insulin infusion[294] and after repeated insulin injections[91] in diabetic patients. In the latter case the deposit was shown to contain intact insulin molecules. Insulin pump therapy has also been shown to be associated with raised serum amyloid A protein[57]. Thus, there seems to be strong evidence that, under certain conditions, insulin fibrils are also formed *in vivo*.

D. CHEMICAL STABILITY

1. Introduction

In contrast to the physical changes in structure, the chemical, covalent changes in the structure are irreversible and may lead to formation of molecules which are less active and potentially immunogenic. Proteins are known to be degraded non-enzymatically by various chemical reactions[202]. The most prevalent of these is deamidation, a reaction in which the side chain amide group in glutaminyl or asparaginyl residues is hydrolyzed to form a free carboxylic acid[121,247]. Insulin contains six such residues, Gln^{A5}, Gln^{A15}, Asn^{A18}, Asn^{A21}, Asn^{B3} and Gln^{B4} (Figure 1). In general, asparagine residues are more labile than glutamine residues[247].

The inactivation of insulin induced by exposure to ultraviolet radiation was observed and studied by several groups already in the first decade of the insulin era[62,99,119,145,183,186,187]. It was later demonstrated that the destruction of the physiological action was due to a first order chemical process (photolysis) involving the cystine and, to less extent, the tyrosine residues[111,169,278,297]. Also radiation by ionizing rays has been shown to inactivate insulin[88,116,145,179,219], although irradiation of frozen insulin has been proposed as a method for its sterilization[285]. The investigations presented in the following have included only insulin that has been stored in the dark.

Chemical deterioration of insulin during storage of pharmaceutical preparations becomes apparent when aged samples are analyzed by disc electrophoresis (Figure 4) or by size exclusion chromatography (SEC) (Figure 5). A two-step HPLC method (SEC-HPLC followed by reverse phase HPLC of the individual peaks from the first run) has been used to demonstrate the formation of hydrolysis as well as minor amounts of higher molecular weight transformation (HMWT) products[44].

Dependent on temperature and formulation, the sum of hydrolysis products (as revealed by disc electrophoresis, Figure 4) and HMWT products accounts for 80-90% of the total chemical degradation of insulin observable by using reverse phase HPLC. However, the remaining transformation products are distributed over more than 10 distinct peaks in the chromatogram[49].

2. Formation of hydrolysis products

Hydrolysis of insulin has been studied during storage of various insulin preparations at different temperatures. Insulin deteriorates rapidly in acid formulations due to extensive deamidation at residue A21[296]. In neutral formulations hydrolysis takes place only at Asn^{B3} and at a substantially reduced rate compared with the acid formulations. The B3 transformation results in

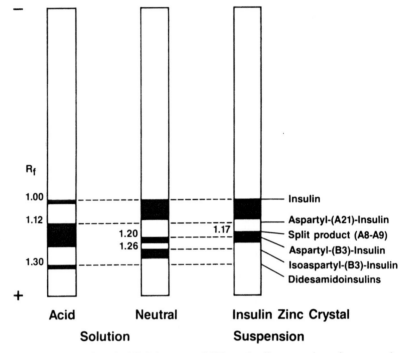

Figure 4. Disc electrophoresis (pH 8.4) pattern of different insulin preparations after storage for 6 months at 25°C. (Adapted from ref. 54 with permission).

formation of a mixture of isoAsp and Asp derivatives[39,43,49]. In the IZS, crystalline (Ultralente) type of preparation an additional hydrolytic reaction leading to main chain cleavage of the A-chain between A8 and A9 is observed[43,49].

a. Deamidation reactions

For 40 years an acid solution of insulin (pH 2–3) was the only rapid acting preparation available. In this formulation monodesamido-(A21)-insulin is formed at a rate of 1–2% per month at 4°C[45]. Stored at 25°C this derivative constitutes more than 90% of the total protein after six months and only small amounts of didesamido derivatives can be observed (Figure 4). If insulin is dissolved in certain diluted mineral acids, e.g. hydrochloric acid, and such solutions are frozen and subsequently thawed, the insulin might be extensively deamidated at Asn^{A2127} due to temporary concentration of the acid. The particular lability of Asn^{A21} towards acid hydrolysis is due to its position as a C-terminal residue, where deamidation is catalyzed by the terminal carboxyl group[7,190]. This special position of one out of three Asn residues in insulin was actually observed before the primary structure of the molecule was known in detail[164].

24

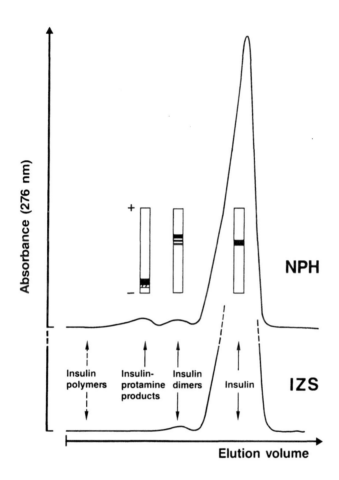

Figure 5. Size exclusion chromatography (SEC) on Biogel P 30 columns of protracted insulin preparations after storage for 12 months at 25°C. Upper panel: Isophane insulin or Neutral Protamine Hagedorn (NPH). Lower panel: Insulin zinc suspension, mixed (IZS). The inserted disc electrophoresis (pH 4) patterns show that the covalent insulin protamine products formed in NPH preparation, and eluting in front of the covalent insulin dimers (CID) on the SEC column, are much more positively charged than the CID. (Adapted from ref. 54 with permission).

In neutral medium insulin deamidates by an entirely different mechanism involving an intermediate formation of a cyclic succinimide at residue B3 which hydrolyzes either under retention of a normal peptide bond B3–B4 (corresponding to simple deamidation) or creation of an isopeptide bond (β-carboxyl linkage). In the latter case the peptide backbone is now directed through the side chain carboxyl group, and the main chain α-carboxyl group is the free acid. The transformation at B3 is independent of concentration (strength) and, except for IZS with crystals, of species of insulin (human, porcine or bovine), but it is strongly influenced by the composition of the neutral solution[49] (Table 3).

The Asn^{B3} deamidation also takes place when insulin is formulated as a suspension with virtually no insulin in solution (<0.1%), but the rate varies with the composition of the medium and the physical state of the insulin (Table 3, Figure 6). In neutral suspensions of amorphously precipitated insulin (i.e. Semilente) deamidation proceeds at the same rate as in neutral solution, but the hydrolysis of the succinimide intermediate now favors formation of the normal Asp derivative which accounts for 65% of the total hydrolysis. The same dominance of the Asp derivative over the isoAsp derivative is observed when neutral suspensions of insulin crystals (i.e. Ultralente or NPH preparations) undergo deamidation, but total deamidation is much slower. Thus deamidation is considerably reduced when the suspended insulin is in the crystalline rather than the amorphous state which indicates that formation of the rate limiting cyclic imide decreases when the flexibility of the tertiary structure is reduced[49]. These results support that tertiary structure is a major determinant to protein deamidation[180,199,292,337].

Deamidation at Asn^{B3} was virtually undetectable in the bovine version of crystalline IZS reflecting the very compact and stable packing of the hexamer in these crystals. In contrast, the porcine and, especially, the human versions of IZS are much more prone to deamidation at Asn^{B3} which might be explained by weaker intermolecular contacts between hexamers in the human insulin crystals[77]. Neutral solutions containing phenol or m-cresol showed lower B3 transformation than the neutral solution with methylparaben as preservative[49]. This is probably due to the stabilizing effect of phenol on the tertiary structure (α-helix formation) around the deamidating residue[87] resulting in reduced probability for imide formation. The phenol-containing crystal suspensions, i.e. NPH and mixtures based on tetragonal crystals, also exhibited relatively low rates of B3 transformation.

The ratio in which the two B3 derivatives (isoAsp/Asp) are formed varies with the formulation, but is independent of time and temperature, suggesting a pathway only involving intermediate imide formation without any direct side chain hydrolysis. In oligopeptides the hydrolytic opening of the intermediate succinimide derivative generates a mixture of deamidated products with an approximately 3:1 predominance of the isoaspartyl residue (i.e. original Asn transformed to isoAsp with a free α-carboxylate group) relative to the normal peptide[64,199,204,210,226,307].

The observed reduction in the isoAsp/Asp ratio when the deamidation takes place in a rigid protein rather than in a conformationally much more flexible peptide[49] (Table 3) is in agreement with findings on deamidation of α-crystallin[316] and of serine hydroxymethyltransferase[11] (ratios 1.6 and 1, respectively).

b. Chain cleavage

In crystalline suspensions containing rhombohedral crystals in combination with a content of surplus zinc ions in addition to the 2–4 structurally bound Zn^{2+} (crystalline and mixed IZS, both with >20 zinc ions/hexamer) cleavage of the

Table 3 Hydrolysis reactions

Preparation	Insulin species	Deamidation (%/month)				Ratio isoAsp/Asp	Chain cleavage A8-A9 (%/month)	
		4°C	15°C	25°C	37°C		4°C	25°C
Regular I	P or H	0.2	0.7	2.1	15	2.0	N.D.	
Regular II	P or H	0.1	0.3	1.1	5.1	1.4	N.D.	
IZS, amorphous	P	0.2	0.8	2.3		0.6	N.D.	
IZS, crystalline	H	0.03		1.0		0.6	< 0.01	0.4
	P	0.02		0.2		0.5	0.01	1.0
	B			< 0.01			0.1	5.9
Isophane (NPH)	H			0.6		0.6	N.D.	
	P			0.3		0.6	N.D.	

The figures are the initial, mean increase of hydrolysis products during storage of insulin preparations (data from ref. 49).
Abbreviations: NPH = Neutral protamine Hagedorn; P = porcine, H = human, B = bovine;
N.D. = not detectable.

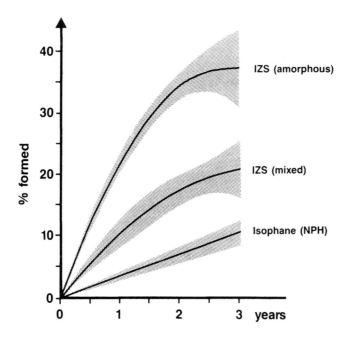

Figure 6. Time courses of formation of the total amounts of hydrolysis products during storage at 25°C of short- and intermediate-acting porcine insulin preparations: Isophane (NPH), and Insulin zinc suspensions (IZS) in two different formulations (mean with 95% confidence interval). (Adapted from ref. 54 with permission).

peptide bond A8–A9 can be observed during normal storage[49]. The rate of formation of this A8–A9 split product is species dependent: Bovine > Porcine > Human insulin. The hydrolytic cleavage of the peptide linkage A8–A9 requires the presence of additional free zinc ions. Thus no cleavage takes place in Biphasic insulin containing the same type of crystal with only 4 zinc ions per hexamer. The main chain hydrolysis is most likely due to an autoproteolytic effect of an adjacent insulin hexamer in the rhombohedral crystal resulting in a metalloproteinase-like cleavage of the peptide chain[52]. The key element for enzyme activity, a Glu carboxylate group is available from the adjacent hexamer, and a zinc ion, supposed to be coordinated to one Glu and two His in the Michaelis complex[303], is available from the medium. In addition, two B5 His residues are in close contact (4 Å) across the hexamer boundary in proximity to the A8 and A9 residues[15], and they actually form a zinc binding site within the crystals[100].

Rate data at 4 and 25°C for these reactions are shown in Table 3. The insulin species variation supports the auto-catalytic theory, as bovine insulin with the fastest formation actually has the closest interactions in the stacking of hexamers in the crystal. The different rate of formation of the split product in bovine insulin relative to human and porcine insulin can also be accounted for by primary structure differences (A8 Ala and Thr, respectively). The slightly faster formation in porcine as compared to human insulin rhombohedral crystals can only be ascribed to differences in the three-dimensional packing of the hexamers in the crystal.

3. Di- and polymerization

Formation of higher molecular weight transformation (HMWT) products during storage of insulin preparations was first reported by Schlichtkrull and coworkers[38,42,43,263]. The main products formed are covalent insulin dimers (CID), but in protamine-containing preparations a concurrent formation of covalent insulin-protamine products (CIPP) takes place at all storage temperatures (Figure 5). At temperatures ≥25°C parallel or consecutive formation of covalent oligomers and polymers can also be observed in certain preparations. CID and CIPP are mainly formed through reactions of amine groups in one molecule with side chain carboxyamide groups in another molecule (transamidation), whereas the formation of polymer is mainly due to chain reactions involving disulfide interactions. Compared with the rate of hydrolysis (see above), rate of HMWT formation is one order of magnitude slower except for NPH preparations, in which the rates (4–25°C) are comparable mainly because of the concomitant formation of CID and CIPP[50] (Table 4).

a. Amine reactions

Rate of CID formation varies with composition and formulation, and for Isophane (NPH) preparations also with the strength of preparation. In neutral solution the rate of CID formation is independent of concentration in the range from U 40 (0.15 mM) to U 500, which strongly indicates that the intermolecular

Table 4 Formation of higher molecular weight transformation products

Type of insulin preparation	Storage temperature (°C)			
	4	15	25	37
		% per year		% per month
Regular I (Human, Porcine)	0.08	0.23	1.0	0.5
Regular II (Human, Porcine)	0.20	0.42	1.3	1.4
IZS, amorphous (porcine)	0.03	0.14	1.0	1.5
IZS, cryst. (Bovine)	0.03	0.24	0.82	1.1
NPH (Human, U 100)	0.5	1.2	3.3	1.6

The figures are the initial, mean increase in the sum of covalent transformation products (covalent insulin dimer, covalent insulin protamine complex and covalent insulin oligo- and polymers) during storage of insulin preparations (data from ref. 50).

chemical reaction occurs mainly within the hexameric units, and not between the hexamers in the solution. As CID formation is of the same order of magnitude in neutral solutions and in suspensions, when these preparations contain the same excipients (Regular I versus IZS types), the covalent insulin dimers in the insulin suspensions most likely also arise from intermolecular reactions within the hexameric unit.

In most types of preparations formation of CID products is only slightly influenced by species of insulin, thus human and porcine insulin exhibit the same stability. During storage at 4°C the most unstable type of preparation is Isophane (NPH) with 15 times faster rate of HMWT formation than the IZS types of preparation. However, at 37°C the transformation in these types of preparation is of the same order of magnitude.

The stability of the neutral solutions is intermediate in this respect, with the glycerol containing Regular II as the most labile. This is in agreement with earlier observations that glycerol in high concentration causes substantially increased formation of covalent insulin di- and polymers[33,38].

In the rhombohedral crystals in IZS,crystalline the trimers and tetramers formed during prolonged storage at temperatures above 25°C are clearly products of consecutive reactions of insulin with already formed insulin dimers and trimers, presumably in the form of successive transamidation[50]. Schlichtkrull[258] observed a prolongation of the timing of action when zinc insulin crystals were heat treated at pH 5.5 ('the thermic effect') and a preparation of this type has been utilized in the treatment of diabetic rats[238]. The prolongation effect can now be explained by cross-links of monomers in the crystals resulting in a reduction of the solubility of such crystals[45].

b. Disulfide interchange reactions

During storage at ambient and higher temperatures, formation of covalent oligomers and polymers can be observed in the neutral solutions and in the preparations containing amorphously precipitated insulin (IZS, amorphous and mixed). These reactions occur in parallel to the formation of dimers, as deduced from the time courses, and are due to disulfide interchange reactions[52]. Such chain reactions may be a result of initial thiol formation through hydrolysis or β-elimination[115,202,220,315]. Intermolecular disulfide exchange requires juxtaposition of disulfide bridges from different insulin molecules. Analyses of the crystal structures by molecular graphics reveal that this is not the case within the hexamer or when hexamers pack in the rhombohedral (IZS crystalline preparations) or monoclinic (NPH) crystals. It is therefore not surprising that covalent polymerization due to disulfide reshuffling is undetectable in these types of preparation even above ambient temperatures. In contrast, disulfide interaction becomes possible when the hexamers approach one another in a random way as in neutral solution or when the insulin is amorphously precipitated[50].

4. Influence of pH and auxiliary substances

The chemical transformation of insulin formulated as Ultralente (Insulin Zinc Suspension, crystalline) as a function of pH is illustrated in Figure 7 A and B. It will appear that there is an optimum for the formation of covalent dimers and oligomers around pH 4 whereas the deterioration due to different hydrolysis reactions is at a minimum around pH 6.5. Similar profiles have been obtained with other types of insulin formulations although in neutral and slightly alkaline media increasing formation of the Asn^{B3} deamidation products with increasing pH can be observed instead of the formation of the A-chain split product seen in the Ultralente crystals[51].

In alkaline media (pH>9) an accelerated formation of covalent oligomers and polymers is seen as a function of pH[51], probably arising as a result of disulfide interactions. Concomitantly lower molecular weight degradation products are formed most likely in the form of insulin A- and B-chains originating from extensive disulfide cleavage by hydrolysis or β-elimination[115].

The types of isotonic substance and preservative have a profound effect on the extent of deamidation as well as on CID formation. There is a clear gradation in the stabilizing effect, for the preservatives: phenol > m-cresol > methylparaben, and for the isotonic agents: NaCl > glycerol > glucose[51]. When used separately the effect of phenol was greater than that of NaCl, but they apparently exert their influence through independent mechanisms as an additive effect was observed by using the two compounds together.

5. Effect of temperature

In all pharmaceutical preparations temperature has a profound influence on the rate of hydrolysis and formation of HMWT-products[49,50,52].

The effect of increasing the temperature by 10°C, coefficient Q_{10}, defined by the expression: $\log Q_{10} = 10 \times (\log k_2 - \log k_1)/(t_2 - t_1)$ with k = rate constant and

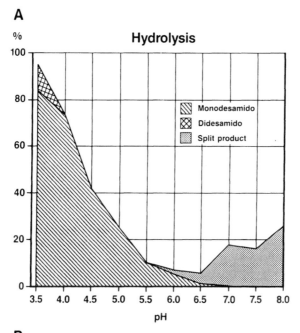

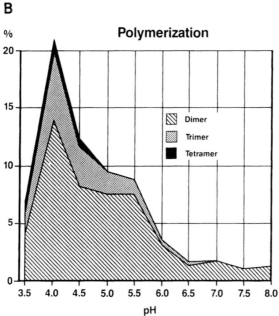

Figure 7. Chemical transformation of insulin during storage of rhombohedral insulin crystals (Bovine insulin crystals, 0.7% NaCl, 0.2% phenol) as a function of pH during storage at 25°C for 12 months. (Adapted from ref. 54 with permission). (A) Formation of the hydrolysis products mono- and didesamido insulins, and the insulin split product (A8–A9). (B) Formation of covalent di- and oligomers.

t=temperature, on the deamidation at Asn^{B3} in the Regular II formulation (pH 7.4) increases with increasing temperature from 2.6 around 10°C to 3.7 around 40°C, reflecting the increase in conformational freedom with increasing temperature.

From the linear parts of the slopes in the Arrhenius plots the activation energy (E_a) for the Asn^{B3} deamidation reaction is calculated to 106 kJ/mol (25.3 kcal/mol) in Regular II (25–45°C). This value is in good agreement with the values of about 22 kcal/mol found under similar conditions for the deamidation of asparaginyl hexapeptides at 30–37°C[121,226].

Temperature has an even more pronounced effect on CID, CIPP and, especially, oligomer and polymer formation. The temperature coefficient Q10 increases from 2–4 at 10°C to 4–16 around 30°C[52].

6. Kinetics and mechanisms

The extreme susceptibility to hydrolysis of the C-terminal residue Asn^{A21} in acid medium, as compared with the other amide groups in insulin, is due to intramolecular catalysis by the protonated C-terminal carboxyl group involving a proton transfer from the COOH-group[190]. After proton transfer to the amide group nucleophilic attack by the carboxylate function forms the cyclic tetrahedral intermediate[172] which after transfer of the proton from the hydroxyl to the nitrogen breaks down to the anhydride by cleavage of the C–N bond, the rate determining step[7,176]. Subsequently the anhydride is readily hydrolysed by general acid catalysis. Alternatively, it has been suggested that the protonated α-carboxylate group stabilizes polarization of the side chain carbomyl group by hydrogen-bonding, which makes the carbon atom more susceptible to hydrolytic attack by solvent nucleophile or to dimerization via transamidation with a terminal amino group[203].

The rate of hydrolysis can be expected to be a function of the degree of protonation of the terminal α-carboxylgroup. In accordance, the rate of A21 deamidation of insulin has been shown to increase with decreasing pH in the pH interval 5 to 2[51]. The additional deamidation of insulin observed from pH 2 to 0.3 can be accounted for by further deamidation by direct hydronium catalyzed amide hydrolysis, not only of Asn^{A21} but also of the other 5 amide groups in insulin, as actually observed[51,296].

The rate determining step in the deamidation reaction at Asn^{B3} in neutral medium is the formation of the intermediate cyclic imide, a much slower process than the subsequent hydrolysis into Asp and isoAsp derivatives[121,210]. The intramolecular imide is hydrolyzed by nucleophilic attack by hydroxide ions, resulting in a mixture of two different desamido products in which the polypeptide backbone is attached via an α-carboxyl linkage (Asp-derivative) or via a β-carboxyl linkage (isoAsp-derivative). Such a mechanism was first proposed to explain the hydrolysis of carbobenzoxy-asparagine derivatives[286] as well as of aspartyl β-ester derivatives[26].

Formation of the succinimide intermediate requires a nucleophilic attack of the main chain peptide nitrogen on the carbonyl carbon of the side chain and this is only possible if these atoms are able to align properly for this reaction. This depends on the side chain bulkiness of the residue on the C-terminal side of the asparaginyl residue[64,121,180,227,247,307] as well as of the three-dimensional conformation and flexibility around the Asn residue[82,180,199,292,337]. Optimal conformation for imide formation occurs when the dihedral torsion angles psi (Ψ) (defining the rotation around the α-carbon/peptide carbonyl carbon bond) is $-120°$[82]. Molecular modelling has shown that succinimide formation at residue B3 requires a more than 100° rotation around the α-carbon/peptide carbonyl carbon which causes an approximately 10 Å movement of the N-terminal B1 residue[52]. This is only possible because the N-terminal residues are on the surface of the insulin hexamer and not very much restricted for such large conformational change.

It is striking that although Asn^{A18} actually has at least as favorable dihedral angles for imide formation as Asn^{B3} [15], no deamidation can be detected in the A-chain at neutral pH[53], probably due to the fact that the A18 residue is part of a helix and therefore with much more reduced conformational flexibility.

If an electronegative side chain, as in the case of the hydroxymethyl group of serine[26,273], is present next to Asn in the sequence or in close proximity in the three dimensional structure, the tendency toward the formation of cyclic intermediates would be enhanced.

The cyclization of the Asn side chain has recently been found to involve pre-equilibrium formation of an anionic intermediate, followed by cyclization and proton transfer to the leaving group from a general acid. The subsequent general-base catalyzed breakdown of the tetrahedral intermediate is the rate-determining step at neutral and basic pH for formation of the succinimide derivative whereas the cyclization step is rate determining at acid pH[65].

The decrease in isoAsp/Asp ratio, observed when the deamidation takes place in a more or less rigid protein rather than in a conformational much more flexible peptide without higher order structural elements, does probably not originate from any direct amide hydrolysis. Instead the reversal in predominance of the individual hydrolytic products may be attributed to variation in local structure around the intermediate imide. Such differences could either result in reduced accessibility to hydrolysis of the succinimide peptide linkage of the imide (isoAsp formation) because of steric hindrance, or increased susceptibility of the imide β-peptide linkage to hydrolysis (Asp formation) due to catalytic effect by juxtaposed functional groups in the three-dimensional structure[52].

CIDs are formed between molecules in the dimeric or hexameric units, common for all types of preparations, mainly through transamidation reactions (aminolysis) by the B-chain N-terminal amine group on Asn side chains of the A-chain[52,142]. A similar intramolecular nucleophilic displacement of an asparaginyl side chain amide by the amino terminus, involving formation of a seven membered cyclic amide, has been described for a tetrapeptide[199].

The independence of CID formation on insulin concentration in the neutral solutions[50] strongly indicates that the intermolecular chemical reaction occurs mainly within the hexameric units and not to any significant extent between the hexamers in the solution. As the crystalline and amorphous suspensions share with the solutions the hexamer as the common unit, it is conceivable that the covalent dimers also mainly form within the hexamer in these preparations. This is supported by the fact that CID formation is of the same order of magnitude in neutral solution and in suspensions when these preparations contain similar auxiliary substances.

In aminolysis of amides an increasing rate of reaction with the acidity of the medium, reaching an essentially constant value below pH 3, has been observed[174]. This is in agreement with our finding that dimer formation (with consecutive transamidation resulting in formation of trimers and tetramers) increases substantially with acidity of the medium from pH 7 to 4[51] (Figure 7B). The steep fall in CID formation from pH 4 to 3.5 most likely reflects the dissociation of the hexamer into mainly dimeric units[35] which gives further evidence for covalent dimer formation primarily being a reaction occurring within the hexamer.

The rate of CID formation is generally faster in glycerol containing preparations, probably due to parallel amine reactions mediated by aldehyde impurities in the glycerol[51]. Aldehydes are able to react chemically with the insulin amino groups through their carbonyl-group under formation of Schiff base adducts. Such reaction products are able to undergo Amadori rearrangement[3] which generates new carbonyl functions capable of forming Schiff base linkages with other amino groups. Eventually such reactions result in covalent crosslinking of the protein[3,22]. Thus, in addition to insulin's potential to form CID by transamidation reactions[52,142], the CID can also be generated via an initial reaction with aldehydes.

It is normally assumed that chemical decomposition of drug suspensions solely takes place in the part of the drug in solution[69]. However, in the IZS types of formulation the amount of insulin in solution is extremely small (<0.1 U/ml). Nevertheless CID forms with the same rate as in the neutral solutions containing 100 U/ml (Table 4), indicating that the transformation reactions in the insulin suspensions mainly takes place within the solid crystalline phase. This is plausible because the hydrated molecules in an insulin crystal show plasticity and have conformational flexibility of their side chains and backbone for movements within the crystal lattice[70,15]. Thus, the switch from extended to the α-helical fold of the N-terminal B-chain segment is accomplished within the crystal lattice although some crystal cracking occurs[25].

CIPP formation probably proceeds via aminolysis by the single amino group (N-terminal) in protamine. Although the content of protamine in the NPH crystals only corresponds to approx. 0.1 protamine molecule per insulin monomer the chemical reaction between protamine and insulin proceeds in the NPH preparation at all temperatures at a rate slightly higher than the rate of insulin dimer formation (Table 4). In NPH (protamine insulin crystals) protamine is situated in the interstices between the hexamers and partly penetrates the central channel of the hexamer. Here it mediates interactions at the dimer-dimer interface but with large conformational flexibility (Dodson, personal comm.). Because of this flexibility of the protamine in the crystals its N-terminal amino group has capacity and possibilities to react with insulin by the same mechanisms as in CID formation.

Formation of covalent polymers in certain formulations at higher storage temperatures can be explained by a chain reaction involving sulfhydryl–disulfide interactions[155,304]. The disulfide in insulin bridging the A7 and B7 residues is on the surface of the hexamer and therefore has the potential to participate in such intermolecular disulfide exchange between hexamers. Such reaction becomes

Table 5 Biological potency of insulin derivatives formed during storage of insulin preparations

Derivative	Preparation isolated from	Insulin species	Bioassay method	Potency relative to insulin
Monodesamido-(A21)-insulin	Acid solution	Porcine	MBG and MCA	92%
		Bovine		85%
Monodesamido-(B3)-insulin	Neutral Regular	Porcine	MCA	97%
Covalent insulin dimer	Insulin Zinc Suspension	Porcine	MBG	15%
Covalent insulin protamine complex	Isophane (NPH)	Bovine	MBG	4%
Covalent insulin polymerization product	Insulin Zinc Suspension (amorphous)	Porcine	MBG	< 2%
Split product (A8–A9)	Insulin Zinc Suspension (crystalline)	Bovine	MBG	2%

The figures are the *in vivo* biological activity relative to an insulin standard (data from ref. 45 and 53).
Abbreviations: MBG = Mouse blood glucose assay; MCA = Mouse convulsion assay.

possible when the individual hexamers are capable of approaching one another in a random way as in solution or when the insulin is amorphously precipitated. An increasing oligomer and polymer formation with increasing insulin concentration in Regular insulin clearly indicates a reaction between the population of hexamers in the neutral solution[50]. Whereas the initial disulfide rupture is a slow process, and therefore rate determining, the subsequent interchange reactions are fast, and as every single interchange leaves a new highly reactive thiolate ion, the initial hydrolysis or β-elimination starts a chain reaction resulting in fast polymer formation. Therefore accumulation of oligomeric disulfide exchange products is insignificant.

7. Properties of transformation products

The different insulin derivatives and higher molecular weight transformation products formed during accelerated storage of insulin preparations have been isolated and characterized with respect to their biological potency and immunogenicity in rabbits[53].

Biological potencies varied from essentially unchanged for the desamido products and down to ≤2% for the A8–A9 split product and the covalent polymerization products (Table 5). The low potency of the split product explains the relatively low biological stability observed during storage of bovine Insulin Zinc Suspension (crystalline)[233].

The immunogenicity (in rabbits) of monodesamido-(A21)- insulin, CID, the covalent insulin polymers[263], monodesamido-(B3)-insulin, CIPP[45] and of the A8–

A9 split product[53] has been found not to be significantly different from the parent insulin.

8. Influence on the quality of pharmaceutical preparations

Among the chemical reactions affecting insulin during storage of the preparations, the hydrolytic reactions dominate and cause transformation of larger amounts of insulin than the di- and polymerization reactions. With respect to the influence on the quality of the insulin preparations, the molecular changes induced by deamidation are relatively small although the isoAsp formation, in addition to changing the uncharged Asn residue into a charged Asp group, also introduces an extra carbon atom into the peptide backbone which may cause more extensive structural changes. However, the deamidation products have essentially the same *in vivo* biological potency as the intact molecule, and also the immunogenicity in rabbits was, as mentioned, unchanged.

Total deamidation during shelf life (2 years) when stored at recommended temperature (2–8°C) is ⩽7%, resulting in insignificant change of the biological potency of the preparations. The cleavage of the peptide backbone of the A-chain between position A8 and A9 represents a much more dramatic change than the deamidation reactions and may induce more serious alterations in the three-dimensional structure of the molecule. In accordance, the *in vivo* potency of the split product is only about 2% of that of the parent hormone (Table 5). However, when the preparations are stored as recommended (temperature interval 2–8°C), the fall in potency during 2 years shelf life is less than 5%[49].

The formation of HMWT products is generally much slower than the chemical decomposition of the insulin due to hydrolytic reactions. The impact on the quality and therapeutical usefulness of the preparations might, however, be more serious as some of the immunological side effects associated with insulin therapy have been asserted to be due to the presence of covalent aggregates of insulin in the therapeutical preparations[240,245,246]. Stored as recommended (2–8°C) the content of CID products at expiry of the preparations is ⩽ 0.5%. In NPH (100 UI/ml) additional formation of CIPP products amounts to ⩽ 0.8%[50].

E. STRUCTURE–STABILITY RELATIONSHIP

It is striking how physical and chemical instability of insulin can be assigned to the domains of the insulin molecule exhibiting the highest degree of conformational flexibility. Thus the predominating physical process leading to precipitation and inactivation of insulin (insulin fibrillation) can be attributed to translocation of the B- chain C-terminal residues, and the dominating chemical degradation of insulin in pharmaceutical formulation, namely deamidation in neutral solution, takes place at the likewise flexible B-chain N-terminal. Also covalent dimerization is mainly mediated via the 'elastic' B1 residue. When addition of phenol or zinc ions constrains the molecules and reduces their flexibility and tendency to disassemble, or if crystal formation renders the molecular assembly more rigid and stable, insulin becomes less prone to fibrillation and chemical degradation.

Summary and conclusion

INTRODUCTION

The present survey deals with the stability aspects of insulin in pharmaceutical formulation and is partly based on the literature and partly on the author's own investigations.

Insulin contains 51 amino acids in two peptide chains (A and B) linked by two disulfide bonds. The A-chain, in addition, contains one internal disulfide bridge. The three- dimensional structure of the insulin molecule (insulin monomer), which is essentially the same in solution and in solid phase, exists in two main conformations. These differ in the extent of α-helix in the B-chain which is influenced by the presence of phenol or its derivatives. In acid and neutral solutions, in concentrations relevant for pharmaceutical formulation, the insulin monomer assembles to dimers and at neutral pH, in the presence of zinc ions, further to hexamers. Many crystalline modifications of insulin have been identified but only those with the hexamer as the basic unit are utilized in preparations for therapy. The insulin hexamer forms a relatively stable unit but some flexibility remains within the individual molecules. The intrinsic flexibility at the ends of the B-chain plays an important role in governing the physical and chemical stability of insulin.

A variety of physical modifications of the secondary to quaternary structures (resulting in 'denaturation', aggregation and precipitation), or chemical changes of the primary structure (yielding insulin derivatives), affect insulin and insulin preparations during handling, storage and use (Figure 8). In the following the experimental results are reviewed and concluded.

PHYSICAL STABILITY

The tendency of insulin, under the influence of heat and exposure to hydrophobic surfaces, to undergo conformational changes resulting in successive, linear aggregation and formation of insoluble insulin fibrils, has been one of the most intriguing and widely studied phenomena in relation to insulin stability. A strong reverse relationship was found between insulin's tendency to fibrillate and its content of insulin related impurities, such as covalent insulin dimer and proinsulin. Insulin fibrillation in neutral solutions of hexameric zinc insulin was demonstrated to be inversely proportional to the concentration of insulin. In contrast, fibrillation in similar solutions of less associated zinc-free

37

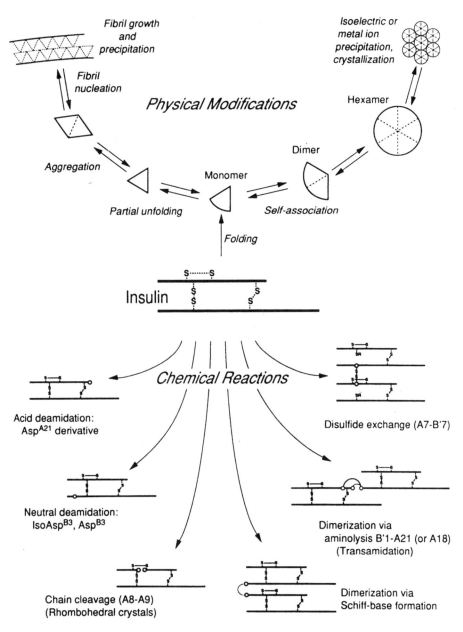

Figure 8. Schematic diagram of the main physical and chemical transformations affecting insulin during storage and use. (Adapted from ref. 54 with permission).

insulin increased with the concentration of insulin, suggesting that formation of fibrils proceeds via monomerization of oligomeric insulin. This would also explain why the presence of hydrophobic interfaces, e.g., liquid/air or liquid/plastic, increases the tendency to fibrillation by inducing dissociation of insulin associates. After monomerization, the initial step in fibril formation seems to be a conformational displacement of 6–8 C-terminal B-chain residues resulting in exposure of certain hydrophobic core residues to the surface of the insulin monomer.

Methods to stabilize insulin solutions against insulin fibrillation include formulation with organic additives like polyols or inorganic additives like certain divalent metal ions. Many of the proposed additives, however, had a deteriorating effect on insulin. Thus addition of certain polysaccharides as well as glycerol caused an unacceptable decrease in the chemical and biological stability of the insulin preparation. The stabilizing effect of polyols seems to correlate with the capacity of these products to react chemically with the insulin amino groups. Hence aldoses were generally more effective than ketoses, and the deteriorating effect of glycerol was related to its content of aldehyde impurities.

Addition of calcium or supplement zinc ions significantly improved the physical stability of neutral insulin solutions, probably by stabilizing the hexameric assembly of insulin molecules. A remarkable stabilizing effect has been obtained by addition of low concentrations of certain detergents, which is a result of their ability to inhibit adsorption of insulin onto hydrophobic surfaces. Extraordinary stabilization was seen when this method was combined with the metal ion stabilization mentioned above.

CHEMICAL STABILITY

Insulin decomposes by a multitude of chemical reactions. Deterioration during storage of pharmaceutical preparations mainly was due to two categories of chemical reactions, hydrolysis, and insulin intermolecular transformation reactions leading to higher molecular weight transformation (HMWT) products. The predominant hydrolysis reaction was deamidation of Asn residues which in acid solution takes place at the A21 residue, in neutral and alkaline medium at the B3 residue. Whereas the acid deamidation at Asn^{A21} was relatively rapid and leads to the normal aspartic acid derivative only, the deamidation reaction at Asn^{B3} was one order of magnitude slower and resulted in formation of a mixture of isoAsp and Asp derivatives. These products result from intermediate formation of a cyclic imide, which hydrolyzes either under retention of a normal peptide bond or an isopeptide bond between B3 and B4. The ratio isoAsp/Asp derivative was independent of time and temperature. However, increasing formation of Asp relative to isoAsp derivative was observed with decreasing flexibility of the insulin three-dimensional structure in the formulation. The rate of deamidation at Asn^{B3} was independent of strength of preparation and in most cases, species of insulin, but varied with storage temperature and formulation.

Total transformation at B3 was considerably reduced when insulin is in crystalline as compared to amorphous or soluble state indicating that formation of the rate limiting cyclic imide decreases when the flexibility of the tertiary structure is reduced. Neutral solutions containing phenol exhibited reduced deamidation due to a stabilizing effect of phenol on the tertiary structure (α-helix formation).

In certain crystalline suspensions an amazing thermolysin-like, autoproteolytic cleavage of the peptide bond A8–A9, presumably catalyzed by an adjacent insulin molecule in a neighbour hexamer, has been identified. The hydrolytic cleavage of the peptide backbone took place only in preparations containing rhombohedral crystals in addition to free zinc ions. The rate of formation of this split product was species dependent: Bovine > Porcine > Human insulin.

Intermolecular chemical reactions occurred in all pharmaceutical insulin formulations but at rates which were generally much slower than those observed for hydrolytic reactions. The main products were covalent insulin dimers (CID), but in protamine-containing preparations a concurrent formation of covalent insulin-protamine products (CIPP) took place. At the temperatures at or above 25°C parallel or consecutive formation of covalent insulin oligomers and polymers could also be observed. The HMWT products were mainly formed via intermolecular aminolysis between N-terminal amine and an amide side chain in the insulin A-chain. The CIDs were apparently formed between molecules within the hexameric unit common for all types of preparations and rate of formation was generally faster in glycerol-containing preparations. Formation of covalent insulin oligomers and polymers, as a result of intermolecular disulfide exchange between different insulin molecules, was observed during storage of neutral solutions and preparations containing amorphously precipitated insulin. The rate of formation of HMWT-products varied with the composition and formulation of the preparations, and, in some cases, with the strength and species of insulin.

Intermolecular, covalent cross-linking of insulin molecules occurred via several mechanisms. The most prominent type of mechanism was aminolysis by the α-amino groups of the N-terminals leading to isopeptide linkages with the A-chain side chain amides. The same type of reaction also resulted in covalent cross-linking of the N-terminal in protamine with insulin. Disulfide exchange reactions led to formation of covalent insulin oligomers and polymers.

The type of excipient has a significant effect on the extent of deamidation as well as formation of HMWT products. There was a clear gradation in the stabilizing effect of the bacteriostatic agents: Phenol > m-cresol > methylparaben, and of the isotonic agents: NaCl > glycerol > glucose. Zinc ions, in amounts that promote association of insulin into hexamers, increased the physical as well as the chemical stability. At pH values below five and above eight insulin degraded relatively fast. At acid pH deamidation at residue A21 and covalent insulin dimerization dominated whereas disulfide reactions leading to covalent polymerization and formation of A- and B-chains prevailed in alkaline medium.

The impact of excipients on the chemical processes seems to be dictated mainly via an influence on insulin three-dimensional structure. Also the effect of physical state of the insulin on the chemical stability was complex suggesting an intricate dependence of intermolecular proximity of involved functional groups. Some reactions are catalytically assisted, intra- or intermolecularly, by insulin functional groups in charged or uncharged form. Therefore, pH, in addition to its potential impact on reaction rate per se, also has an effect on insulin charge and, thereby, on folding and association of the insulin molecules. Optimal over-all stability was observed in the pH range 6–7.

In neutral insulin preparations deamidation during shelf life was $\leqslant 7\%$, highest in solutions and amorphous suspensions. Formation of the A8–A9 split product in suspensions containing rhombohedral crystals was $\leqslant 5\%$ in bovine, and at least a factor 10 lower in human insulin preparations. The content of covalent insulin dimers at expiry of the preparations was $\leqslant 0.5\%$. In NPH additional formation of CIPP amounted to $\leqslant 0.8\%$.

CONCLUSION

The stability of insulin in pharmaceutical preparations is, in a very complex manner, dependent on the exact formulation of the product. In modern insulin preparations formulated at neutral pH, and stored as recommended at 2–8°C, less than 10% transformation and degradation products will be formed during shelf life. Formation of the potentially immunogenic covalent higher molecular products will be less than 2%.

The present studies have shown that segmental, conformational flexibility within the insulin molecule is a major determinant controlling the rate of spontaneous structural transformation, and plays a crucial role in insulin stability. Thus, physical as well as chemical deterioration of insulin is almost entirely governed by the capacity of the B-chain terminals to undergo the structural changes necessary for the physical interactions or the chemical reactions to take place.

Resumé og konklusion

INDLEDNING

Nærværende afhandling, der er skrevet som en oversigt over temaet 'insulins stabilitet', er dels en historisk og litteraturmæssig gennemgang af emnet dels et sammendrag og samlet diskussion af en række tidligere offentliggjorte arbejder omhandlende stabilitet af insulin i farmaceutisk formulering.

Insulin er opbygget af 51 aminosyrer i 2 peptidkæder (A og B), som er forbundet med 2 disulfidbroer. A-kæden indeholder desuden en intern disulfidbro. Den tredimensionale struktur af insulinmolekylet (insulinmonomeren), som stort set er ens i opløsning og fast fase (amorf eller krystallinsk form), kan antage to forskellige konformationer. Disse adskiller sig ved omfanget af α-helix i B-kæden, som øges såfremt fenol (eller fenol derivater) er tilstede. Ved insulin koncentrationer, som er relevante for farmaceutisk formulering, associerer insulinmonomerene til insulindimerer i såvel sur som neutral til svagt basisk opløsning. Under tilstedeværelsen af zinkioner vil 3 dimerer i neutralt til svagt surt medium yderligere associere til en insulinhexamer. Insulin er i stand til at krystallisere i en lang række forskellige modifikationer, men kun sådanne som baserer sig på insulinhexameren bliver anvendt i farmaceutiske præparater. Insulinhexameren udgør en relativt stabil enhed, hvor dog nogen fleksibilitet af peptidkæden er bevaret indenfor det enkelte molekyle i opløsning såvel som i krystaller. Dette gælder specielt begge ender af B-kæden, og som det vil fremgå af det følgende spiller dette forhold en vigtig rolle for insulins fysiske og kemiske stabilitet.

En række fysiske modifikationer af insulins sekundære til kvaternære struktur (resulterende i 'denaturering', aggregatdannelse og udfældning) eller kemiske ændringer af den primære struktur (derivatdannelse) kan påvirke insulinstrukturen i forbindelse med håndtering, opbevaring eller brug (se figur 8). I det følgende bliver de eksperimentelle resultater resumeret og konkluderet.

FYSISK STABILITET

Når insulin opløsninger udsættes for varme kombineret med hydrofobe overflader, har insulinet en tendens til ændring af den native, rumlige struktur med efterfølgende lineær aggregering af insulinmolekyler gennem hydrofobe interaktioner. Dette fører til udfældning af fibrillignende produkter, og denne egenskab ved insulinet har været et af de mest undersøgte stabilitetsfænomener.

Tendensen til fibrillering af insulin er omvendt proportional med indholdet af insulinlignende urenheder såsom covalent insulindimer og proinsulin. I neutrale opløsninger af hexamert zink-insulin stiger tendensen til fibrillering, når koncentrationen af insulin falder. Det omvendte er tilfældet når opløsningen indeholder mindre associeret, zinkfrit insulin. Og da ydermere fibrillerings tendensen stiger med tiltagende dissociering, indicerer dette, at den initiale strukturændring fordrer en monomerisering af insulinet. Dette forklarer også, hvorfor tilstedeværelsen af hydrofobe grænseflader, f.eks. luft/opløsning eller plast/opløsning, fremskynder fibrillering af insulinet ved at fremme dissociering af de associerede insulin molekyler. Efter monomeriseringen indledes fibrildannelsesprocessen med en ændring af konformationen af de sidste 6-8 aminosyre enheder i B-kædens N-terminal, som medfører en blotlægning af visse af de hydrofobe områder, som ellers er gemt i monomerens indre.

Metoder til at stabilisere insulin opløsninger imod fibrillering inkluderer tilsætning af en række organiske additiver, såsom polyalkoholforbindelser, eller uorganiske additiver, såsom divalente metalioner. Mange af disse additiver har en nedbrydende effekt på insulinet, f.eks. ødelægger visse kulhydrater såvel som glycerol den kemiske og biologiske stabilitet af insulinpræparatet. Den stabiliserende effekt af polyalkoholerne synes at korrelere med deres evne til at reagere kemisk med insulinets aminogrupper. Således er aldoser generelt mere effektive end ketoser, og effekten af glycerol er relateret til dets indhold af aldehyd urenheder. Tilsætning af calcium- eller zink-ioner giver en væsentlig forbedring af neutrale insulinopløsningers fysiske stabilitet. Den gode effekt skyldes sandsynligvis at metalionerne neutraliserer negative ladninger i insulin hexamerens centrum og dermed stabiliserer denne. En bemærkelsesværdig stabilisering opnås med lave koncentrationer af visse detergenter, hvilket kan forklares med at disse hæmmer insulinets adsorption til hydrofobe overflader. Særlig god fysisk stabilisering opnås med en kombination af detergent- og metalionadditiver.

KEMISK STABILITET

En lang række forskellige kemiske reaktioner medvirker til at omdanne insulin. Nedbrydning under lagring af insulinpræparater kan især henføres til to typer af kemiske reaktioner, nemlig hydrolyse samt inter-molekylære reaktioner. Sidstnævnte reaktionstype fører til produkter med højere molvægt (HMV) herunder covalente insulindimerer (CID) og polymerisationsprodukter. Den dominerende hydrolysereaktion viste sig at være deamidering af asparagin-grupper. Tidligere arbejder har vist at deamidering ved sur reaktion finder sted i Asn^{A21}, mens nærværende studier har påvist at den ved neutral til svagt basisk reaktion foregår i Asn^{B3}. Mens den sure deamidering af Asn^{A21}, som foregår relativt hurtigt, kun førte til det normale asparaginsyrederivat, så dannedes der ved den noget langsommere, neutrale deamidering såvel Asp^{B3}- som $isoAsp^{B3}$-insulin. Dette foregår via en indledende dannelse af et cyklisk imid, som efterfølgende hurtigt hydrolyserer delvist på den ene delvist på den anden side af imid- nitrogenatomet. Dermed genoprettes der dels en normal peptidbinding (Asp-derivat), dels etableres der en β-peptidbinding (isoAsp-derivat) mellem B3 og B4. Forholdet isoAsp/Asp var uafhængig af tid og temperatur, men der sås øget dannelse af Asp-derivatet relativt til isoAsp-derivatet når fleksibiliteten af insulinets tredimensionale struktur var øget i den pågældende formulering. Deamideringshastigheden af Asn^{B3} var uafhængig af præparatets styrke og som hovedregel også oprindelsen (dyrearten) af insulinet, men varierede med temperaturen og med formuleringen af det pågældende præparat.

Med insulinet i krystallinsk form var omdannelsen af Asn^{B3} væsentligt reduceret i sammenligning med insulin i amorf eller opløst form. Dette indicerer, at dannelsen af det cykliske imid, som er hastighedsbestemmende for totalreaktionen, mindskes, når fleksibiliteten af den tertiære struktur nedsættes. Neutrale opløsninger med indhold af fenol udviste reduceret deamidering, hviket må tilskrives fenolens stabiliserende indflydelse på strukturen af hexameren (α-helix dannelse).

En forbløffende termolysin-lignende, autoprotolytisk spaltning af A8–A9 peptidbindingen blev iagttaget i visse krystallinske præparater. Reaktionen er formodentlig katalyseret af et tilstødende insulinmolekyle i en nabo hexamer. Den hydrolytiske spaltning af peptidkæden fandt kun sted i præparater som indeholdt rhomboedriske krystaller og ydermere kun, når der var frie zinkioner tilstede i opløsningen. Dannelsen af dette splitprodukt var dyreart afhængig: Okse > Svine > Human insulin.

Intermolekylære kemiske reaktioner fandt sted i alle præparater, men hastigheden, hvormed produkterne dannedes, var generelt væsentligt lavere end for de hydrolytiske reaktioner. Hovedprodukterne bestod af CID, men sideløbende dannedes der covalente insulin-protaminprodukter (CIPP) i præparater med indhold af protamin. Parallelt eller konsekutivt forløbende dannelse af covalente insulinoligo- eller polymere sås ved opbevaringstemperaturer ≥ 25°C. Dannelsen af HMV-produkterne kan hovedsagelig henføres til intermolekylær aminolyse mellem en N-terminal amin og en amid sidekæde i insulinets A-kæde. CID-produkterne blev tilsyneladende dannet mellem molekyler indenfor hexameren, en fælles enhed for alle neutrale insulinpræparater, og dannelseshastigheden var generelt større når præparatet indeholdt glycerol. Dannelsen af covalente insulinoligo- og polymere, som et resultat af intermolekylære disulfid-interaktioner, sås i præparater med insulin i opløst eller amorft udfældet form. Dannelseshastigheden for HMV-produkterne varierede med kompositionen og formuleringen af præparaterne og i enkelte tilfælde også med styrken samt dyrearten af insulinet.

Hjælpestofferne har en væsentlig indflydelse på graden af deamidering såvel som dannelse af HMV-produkterne. Der var således en klar graduering af den stabiliserende effekt af konserveringsmidler (fenol > m-kresol > metyl-p-hydroxybenzosyre) og af isotonika (natriumklorid > glycerol > glukose). Zinkioner havde, i mængder som deltager i dannelsen af insulinhexameren, både fysisk og kemisk en stabiliserende effekt.

Insulin nedbrydes relativt hurtigt ved pH-værdier under 5 og over 8. Ved sur reaktion dominerede A21 deamidering samt CID-dannelse, hvorimod disulfidreaktioner, som dels leder til polymerisation og dels til adskillelse i A- og B-kæder, var mest fremtrædende i basisk medium.

Hjælpestoffer og pH har således en ret kompleks indflydelse, men en fælles faktor i forbindelse med hydrolyse- såvel som de intermolekylære tværbindingsreaktioner synes at være deres effekt på konformationen rundt om reaktanterne. Nogle af reaktionerne er intra- eller intermolekylært katalyseret af insulinets funktionelle grupper i ladet eller uladet form. Udover effekten af pH-værdien på reaktionshastigheden per se har den også indflydelse på insulinets ladningsforhold og dermed på lokal konformation samt associeringsforhold. Optimal stabilitet sås i pH-området 6–7.

Intermolekylær tværbinding af insulinmolekyler kan forgå ved flere forskellige mekanismer. Den dominerende reaktion er aminolyse af sidekæde amidgrupper i A-kæden forårsaget af α-aminogruppen i en af de to N-terminaler. Reaktionen fører til isopeptidbindinger, hvilket på samme vis kan opstå mellem insulin og N-teminalen i protamin. Disulfidinteraktioner resulterer i en kædereaktion som fører til insulinoligomere og -polymere. I neutrale insulin præparater var deamideringen størst i opløsninger samt amorfe suspensioner, men udgjorde dog ved præparaternes udløb mindre end 7%. Dannelsen af det biologisk nærmest inaktive A8–A9 splitprodukt i suspensioner med okse insulinkrystaller nåede i samme tidsrum op på ca. 5%, mens det var mindst en ti-faktor lavere for human insulin. Indholdet af CID var ved udløb $\leqslant 0.5\%$. I NPH-præparater vil den sideløbende dannelse af CIPP udgøre $\leqslant 0.8\%$.

KONKLUSION

Stabiliteten af insulin i farmaceutiske præparater er på kompliceret vis påvirket af den eksakte formulering af produktet. I insulinpræparater formuleret ved neutral pH og opbevaret som foreskrevet ved 2–8°C, vil der ved udløb være dannet mindre end 10% omdannelsesprodukter. Dannelsen af potentielt immunogene højere-molvægts-produkter vil i løbetiden udgøre mindre end 2%. De foreliggende studier har klart vist, at fleksibilitet af lokale konformationer i insulin strukturen spiller en afgørende rolle for insulinets stabilitet. Således er både den fysiske og kemiske omdannelse af insulin nærmest fuldstændig bestemt af evnen af B-kædens to ender til at undergå strukturmæssige ændringer.

References
(references from submitted papers included)

1. Abel, J.J. Crystalline insulin. *Proc.Natl.Acad.Sci.USA* 12:132-136, 1926.
2. Abel, J.J. and Geiling, E.M.K. Researches on insulin. I. Is insulin an unstable sulphur compound? *J.Pharmacol.Exp.Ther.* 25:423-448, 1925.
3. Acharya, A.S. and Manning, J.M. Reaction of glycolaldehyde with proteins: Latent crosslinking potential of α-hydroxyaldehydes. *Proc.Natl.Acad.Sci.USA* 80:3590-3594, 1983.
4. Adams, M.J., Blundell, T.L., Dodson, E.J., Dodson, G.G., Vijayan, M., Baker, E.N., Harding, M.M., Hodgkin, D.C., Rimmer, B. and Sheat, S. Structure of rhombohedral 2 zinc insulin crystals. *Nature* 224:491-495, 1969.
5. Albisser, A.M., Lougheed, W.D., Perlman, K. and Bahoric, A. Nonaggregating insulin solutions for long-term glucose control in experimental and human diabetes. *Diabetes* 29:241-243, 1980.
6. Albisser, A.M., Williamson, J.R. and Lougheed, W.D. Desired characteristics of insulins to be used in infusion pumps. In: *Hormone Drugs*, edited by Gueriguian, J.L., Bransome, E.D. and Outschoorn, A.S. Rockville: United States Pharmacopeial Convention, 1982, p. 84-95.
7. Aldersley, M.F., Kirby, A.J., Lancaster, P.W., McDonald, R.S. and Smith, C.R. Intramolecular catalysis of amide hydrolysis by the carboxy-group. Rate determining proton transfer from external general acids in the hydrolysis of substituted maleamic acids. *J.Chem.Soc.Perkin Trans.* 2:1487-1495, 1974.
8. Ambrose, E.J. and Elliott, A. Infra-red spectroscopic studies of globular protein structure. *Proc.Royal Soc.(London)* 208:75-90, 1951.
9. Ansari, A., Jones, C.M., Henry, E.C., Hofrichter, J. and Eaton, W.A. The role of solvent viscosity in the dynamics of protein conformational changes. *Science* 256:1796-1798, 1992.
10. Arakawa, T. and Timasheff, S.N. Stabilization of protein structure by sugars. *Biochemistry* 21:6536-6544, 1982.
11. Artigues, A., Birkett, A. and Schirch, V. Evidence for the in vivo deamidation and isomerization of an asparaginyl residue in cytosolic serine hydroxymethyltransferase. *J.Biol.Chem.* 265:4853-4858, 1990.
12. Aswad, D.W. Stoichiometric methylation of porcine adrenocorticotropin by protein carboxyl methyltransferase requires deamidation of asparagine 25. Evidence for methylation at the α-carboxyl group of atypical l-isoaspartyl residues. *J.Biol.Chem.* 259:10714-10721, 1984.
13. Back, J.F., Oakenfull, D. and Smith, M.B. Increased thermal stability of proteins in the presence of sugars and polyols. *Biochemistry* 18:5191-5196, 1979.
14. Baker, E.N. and Dodson, G. X-ray diffraction data on some crystalline varieties of insulin. *J.Mol.Biol.* 54:605-609, 1970.
15. Baker, E.N., Blundell, T.L., Cutfield, J.F., Cutfield, S.M., Dodson, E.J., Dodson, G.G., Hodgkin, D.M.C., Hubbard, R.E., Isaacs, N.W., Reynolds, C.D., Sakabe, K., Sakabe, N. and Vijayan, N.M. The structure of 2Zn pig insulin crystals at 1.5 Å resolution. *Phil.Trans.R.Soc.* 319:369-456, 1988.
16. Balschmidt, P., Hansen, F.B., Dodson, E.J., Dodson, G.G. and Korber, F. Structure of porcine insulin cocrystallized with clupeine Z. *Acta Cryst.* B47:975-986, 1991.
17. Banting, F.G. and Best, C.H. The internal secretion of the pancreas. *J.Lab.Clin.Med.* 7:251-266, 1921.
18. Banting, F.G. and Best, C.H. Pancreatic extracts. *J.Lab.Clin.Med.* 7:464-472, 1922.

19. Banting, F.G., Best, C.H., Collip, J.B. and Macleod, J.J.R. The preparation of pancreatic extracts containing insulin. *Trans.R.S.C.* 16:27-29, 1922.
20. Barber, J.R. and Clarke, S. Demethylation of protein carboxyl methyl esters: A nonenzymatic process in human erythrocytes. *Biochemistry* 24:4867-4871, 1985.
21. Battersby, A.R. and Robinson, J.C. Studies on specific chemical fission of peptide links. Part I. The rearrangement of aspartyl and glutamyl peptides. *J.Biol.Chem.* 246:259-269, 1955.
22. Bello, J. and Bello, H.R. Chemical modification and cross-linking of proteins by impurities in glycerol. *Arch.Biochem.Biophys.* 172:608-610, 1976.
23. Bender, M.L. General acid-base catalysis in the intramolecular hydrolysis of phthalamic acid. *J.Am.Chem.Soc.* 79:1258-1259, 1957.
24. Bender, M.L. and Neveu, M.C. Intramolecular catalysis of hydrolytic reactions. IV. A comparison of intramolecular and intermolecular catalysis. *J.Am.Chem.Soc.* 80:5388-5391, 1958.
25. Bentley, G., Dodson, G. and Lewitova, A. Rhombohedral insulin crystal transformation. *J.Mol.Biol.* 126:871-875, 1978.
26. Bernhard, S.A., Berger, A., Carter, J.H., Katchalski, E., Sela, M. and Shalitin, Y. Co-operative effects of functional groups in peptides. I. Aspartyl-serine derivatives. *J.Am.Chem.Soc.* 84:2421-2434, 1962.
27. Berson, S.A. and Yalow, R.S. Deamidation of insulin during storage in frozen state. *Diabetes* 15:875-879, 1966.
28. Best, C.H. and Macleod, J.J.R. Some chemical reactions of insulin. *J.Biol.Chem.* 55:29-30, 1923.
29. Bhatt, N.P., Patel, K. and Borchardt, R.T. Chemical pathways of peptide degradation. I. Deamidation of adrenocorticotropic hormone. *Pharm.Res.* 7:593-599, 1990.
30. Bi, R.C., Dauter, Z., Dodson, E., Dodson, G., Giordano, F. and Reynolds, C. Insulin's structure as a modified and monomeric molecule. *Biopolymers* 23:391-395, 1984.
31. Binder, C. A theoretical model for the absorption of soluble insulin. In: *Artificial Systems for Insulin Delivery*, edited by Brunetti, P., Alberti, K.G.M.M., Albisser, A.M., Hepp, K.D. and Benedetti, M.M. New York: Raven Press, 1983, p. 53-57.
32. Bischoff, F. and Sahyun, M. Denaturation of insulin protein by concentrated sulfuric acid. *J.Biol.Chem.* 81:167-173, 1929.
33. Blackshear, P.J., Rohde, T.D., Palmer, J.L., Wigness, B.D., Rupp, W.M. and Buchwald, H. Glycerol prevents insulin precipitation and interruption of flow in an implantable insulin infusion pump. *Diabetes Care* 6:387-392, 1983.
34. Blatherwick, N.R., Bischoff, F., Maxwell, L.C., Berger, J. and Sahyun, M. Studies on insulin. *J.Biol.Chem.* 72:57-89, 1927.
35. Blundell, T., Dodson, G., Hodgkin, D. and Mercola, D. Insulin: The structure in the crystal and its reflection in chemistry and biology. *Adv.Protein Chem.* 26:279-402, 1972.
36. Bornstein, P. and Balian, G. The specific nonenzymatic cleavage of bovine ribonuclease with hydoxylamine. *J.Biol.Chem.* 245:4854-4856, 1970.
37. Brand, E. and Sandberg, M. The lability of the sulfur in cystine derivatives and its possible bearing on the constitution of insulin. *J.Biol.Chem.* 70:381-395, 1926.
38. Brange, J., Havelund, S., Hansen, P., Langkjaer, L., Sørensen, E. and Hildebrandt, P. Formulation of physically stable neutral solutions for continuous infusion by delivery systems. In: *Hormone Drugs*, edited by Gueriguian, J.L., Bransome, E.D. and Outschoorn, A.S. Rockville, MD: US Pharmacopoeial Convention, 1982, p. 96-105.
39. Brange, J. and Havelund, S. Properties of insulin in solution. In: *Artificial systems for insulin delivery*, edited by Brunetti, P., Alberti, K.G.M.M., Albisser, A.M., Hepp, K.D. and Benedetti, M.M. New York: Raven Press, 1983, p. 83-88.
40. Brange, J. and Havelund, S. Insulin pumps and insulin quality – Requirements and problems. *Acta Med.Scand.* 671 (Suppl.):135-138, 1983.
41. Brange, J., Langkjaer, L., Havelund, S. and Sørensen, E. Chemical stability of insulin: Neutral insulin solutions. *Diabetologia* 25:193, 1983.
42. Brange, J., Langkjaer, L., Havelund, S. and Sørensen, E. Chemical stability of insulin: Formation of covalent insulin dimers and other higher molecular weight transformation products in intermediate- and long-acting insulin preparations. *Diabetologia* 27:259-260, 1984.(Abstract)
43. Brange, J., Langkjaer, L., Havelund, S. and Sørensen, E. Chemical stability of insulin: Formation of desamido insulins and other hydrolytic products in intermediate- and long-acting insulin preparations. *Diabetes Res.Clin.Pract.* 1 (Suppl.):67, 1985.(Abstract)

44. Brange, J., Havelund, S., Hommel, E., Sørensen, E. and Kühl, C. Neutral insulin solutions physically stabilized by addition of Zn^{2+}. *Diabetic Med.* 3:532-536, 1986.
45. Brange, J., Skelbaek-Pedersen, B., Langkjaer, L., Damgaard, U., Ege, H., Havelund, S., Heding, L.G., Jørgensen, K.H., Lykkeberg, J., Markussen, J., Pingel, M. and Rasmussen, E. *Galenics of Insulin: The Physico-chemical and Pharmaceutical Aspects of Insulin and Insulin Preparations,* Berlin, Heidelberg, New York, London, Paris, Tokyo: Springer-Verlag, 1987.
46. Brange, J., Hansen, J.F., Havelund, S. and Melberg, S.G. Studies of the insulin fibrillation process. In: *Advanced Models for the Therapy of Insulin-Dependent Diabetes,* edited by Brunetti, P. and Waldhäusl, W.K. New York: Raven Press, 1987, p. 85-90.
47. Brange, J., Ribel, U., Hansen, J.F., Dodson, G., Hansen, M.T., Havelund, S., Melberg, S.G., Norris, F., Norris, K., Snel, L., Sørensen, A.R. and Voigt, H.O. Monomeric insulins obtained by protein engineering and their medical implications. *Nature* 333:679-682, 1988.
48. Brange, J., Owens, D.R., Kang, S. and Vølund, A. Monomeric insulins, and their experimental and clinical implications. *Diabetes Care* 13:923-954, 1990.
49. Brange, J., Langkjær, L., Havelund, S. and Vølund, A. Chemical stability of insulin: 1. Hydrolytic degradation during storage of pharmaceutical preparations. *Pharm.Res.* 9:715-726, 1992.
50. Brange, J., Havelund, S. and Hougaard, P. Chemical stability of insulin: 2. Formation of higher molecular weight transformation products during storage of pharmaceutical insulin preparations. *Pharm.Res.* 9:727-734, 1992.
51. Brange, J. and Langkjær, L. Chemical stability of insulin: 3. Influence of excipients, formulation, and pH. *Acta Pharm.Nord.* 4:149-158, 1992.
52. Brange, J. Chemical stability of insulin: 4. Kinetics and mechanisms of the chemical transformation in pharmaceutical formulation. *Acta Pharm.Nord.* 4:209-222, 1992.
53. Brange, J., Hallund, O. and Sørensen, E. Chemical stability of insulin: 5. Isolation, characterization and identification of insulin transformation products. *Acta Pharm.Nord.* 4:223-232, 1992.
54. Brange, J. and Langkjær, L. Insulin structure and stability. In: *Stability and Characterization of Protein and Peptide Drugs: Case Histories,* edited by Wang, Y.J. and Pearlman, R. New York: Plenum Press, 1993, p. 315-350.
55. Brennan, J.R., Gebhart, S.P. and Blackard, W.G. Pump-induced insulin aggregation. A problem with the Biostator. *Diabetes* 34:353-359, 1985.
56. Bringer, J., Heldt, A. and Grodsky, G.M. Prevention of insulin aggregation by dicarboxylic amino acids during prolonged infusion. *Diabetes* 30:83-85, 1981.
57. Brownlee, M., Cerami, A., Li, J.J., Vlassara, H., Martin, T.R. and McAdam, K.P.W.J. Association of insulin pump therapy with raised serum amyloid A in type I diabetes mellitus. *Lancet* 1:411-413, 1984.
58. Bruch, E. Über kristallinisches Insulin. 11. Mitteilung: Darstellung und chemische Eigenschaften. *Arch.Exper.Path.Pharmakol.* 173:439-451, 1933.
59. Bruice, T.C. and Pandit, U.K. The effect of geminal substitution ring size and rotamer distribution on the intramolecular nucleophilic catalysis of the hydrolysis of monophenyl esters of dibasic acids and the solvolysis of the intermediate anhydrides. *J.Am.Chem.Soc.* 82:5858-5865, 1960.
60. Buchwald, H., Rohde, T.D., Dorman, F.D., Skakoon, J.G., Wigness, B.D., Prosl, F.R., Tucker, E.M., Rublein, T.G., Blackshear, P.J. and Varco, R.L. A totally implantable drug infusion device: Laboratory and clinical experience using a model with single flow rate and new design for modulated insulin infusion. *Diabetes Care* 3:351-358, 1980.
61. Buchwald, H., Varco, R.L., Rupp, R.L., Goldenberg, F.J., Barbosa, J., Rohde, T.D., Schwartz, R.A., Rublein, T.G. and Blackshear, P.J. Treatment of a type II diabetic by a totally implantable insulin infusion device. *Lancet* 1:1233-1235, 1981.
62. Burge, W.E. and Wickwire, G.C. The decrease in sugar metabolism and destruction of insulin by ultra-violet radiation. *J.Biol.Chem.* 72:827-831, 1927.
63. Burke, M.J. and Rougvie, M.A. Cross-β protein structures. I. Insulin fibrils. *Biochemistry* 11:2435-2439, 1972.
64. Capasso, S., Mazzarella, L., Sica, F. and Zagari, A. Deamidation via cyclic imide in asparaginyl peptides. *Peptide Research* 2:195-200, 1989.
65. Capasso, S., Mazzarella, L., Sica, F., Zagari, A. and Salvadori, S. Kinetics and mechanism of succinimide ring formation in the deamidation process of asparagine residues. *J.Chem.Soc.,Perkin Trans.* 2:679-682, 1993.

66. Carlson, G.A., Bair, R.E., Gaona, J.I.,Jr., Love, J.T., Schildknecht, H.E., Urenda, R.S., Spencer, W.J., Eaton, R.P. and Schade, D.S. An implantable, remotely programmable insulin infusion system. *Med.Progr.Technol.* 9:17-25, 1982.
67. Carpenter, F.H. Relationship of structure to biological activity of insulin as revealed by degradative studies. *Am.J.Med.* 40:750-758, 1966.
68. Carr, F.H., Culhane, K., Fuller, A.T. and Underhill, S.W.F. A reversible inactivation of insulin. *Biochem.J.* 23:1010-1021, 1929.
69. Carstensen, J.T. *Drug stability: Principles and practices*, New York, Basel:Dekker, 1990.
70. Caspar, D.L.D. and Badger, J. Plasticity of crystalline proteins. *Current Opinion in Structural Biology* 1:877-882, 1991.
71. Cavallini, D., Federici, G. and Barboni, E. Interaction of protein with sulfide. *Eur.J.Biochem.* 14:169-174, 1970.
72. Cecil, R. and McPhee, J.R. The sulfur chemistry of proteins. *Adv.Protein Chem.* 14:255-389, 1959.
73. Cecil, R. and Loening, U.E. The reactions of the disulphide groups of insulin with sodium sulphite. *Biochem.J.* 76:146-155, 1960.
74. Champion, M.C., Shepherd, G.A.A., Rodger, N.W. and Dupre, J. Continuous subcutaneous infusion of insulin in the management of diabetes mellitus. *Diabetes* 29:206-212, 1980.
75. Chance, R.E. Amino acid sequences of proinsulins and intermediates. *Diabetes* 21 (Suppl. 2):461-467, 1972.
76. Charles, A.F. and Scott, D.A. Action of acid alcohol on insulin. *J.Biol.Chem.* 92:289-302, 1931.
77. Chawdhury, S.A., Dodson, E.J., Dodson, G.G., Reynolds, C.D., Tolley, S.P., Blundell, T.L., Cleasby, A., Pitts, J.E., Tickle, I.J. and Wood, S.P. The crystal structure of three non-pancreatic human insulins. *Diabetologia* 25:460-464, 1983.
78. Chawla, A.S., Hinberg, I., Blais, P. and Johnson, D. Aggregation of insulin, containing surfactants, in contacts with different materials. *Diabetes* 34:420-424, 1985.
79. Chazin, W.J., Kördel, J., Thulin, E., Hofmann, T., Drakenberg, T. and Forsén, S. Identification of an isoaspartyl linkage formed upon deamidation of bovine calbindin D9k and structural characterization by 2D 1H NMR. *Biochemistry* 28:8646-8653, 1989.
80. Cheadle, F.M. Studies on insulin, II. The effect of hydrogen-ion concentration on the activity of insulin subjected to high temperatures. *Aust.J.Exp.Biol.* 1:129-130, 1924.
81. Choay, A. Sur la conservation de L'insuline. *Comptes Rendue Soc.Biologie* 94:178-180, 1926.
82. Clarke, S. Propensity for spontaneous succinimide formation from aspartyl and asparaginyl residues in cellular proteins. *Int.J.Peptide Protein Res.* 30:808-821, 1987.
83. Cohen, A.S. and Calkins, E. Electron microscopic observations on a fibrous component in amyloid of diverse origins. *Nature* 183:1202-1203, 1959.
84. Csorba, T.R., Gattner, H.G. and Cuatrecasas, P. Partial dimerization of insulin. *Clin.Res.* 20:918, 1972.(Abstract)
85. Dahlgren, G. and Simmerman, N.L. The effect of ethyl substitution on the kinetics of the hydrolysis of maleamic and phthalamic acid. *J.Phys.Chem.* 69:3626-3630, 1965.
86. Dathe, M., Gast K., Zirwer, D., Welfle, H. and Mehlis, B. Insulin aggregation in solution. *Int.J.Peptide Protein Res.* 36:344-349, 1990.
87. Derewenda, U., Derewenda, Z., Dodson, E., Dodson, G.G., Reynolds, C.D., Smith, G.D., Sparks, C. and Swenson, D. Phenol stabilizes more helix in a new symmetrical zinc insulin hexamer. *Nature* 338:594-596, 1989.
88. Desai, A.M. and Korgaonkar, K.S. Studies on the effects of cobalt-60 gamma rays on protamine sulfate, lysozyme and insulin by using monolayer technique. *Radiation Res.* 21:61-74, 1964.
89. Diaugustini, R.P., Gibson, B.W., Aberth, W., Kelly, M., Ferrua, C.M., Tomooka, Y., Brown, C.F. and Walker, M. Evidence for isoaspartyl (deamidated) forms of mouse epidermal growth factor. *Anal.Biochem.* 165:420-429, 1987.
90. Dickens, F., Dodds, E.C., Lawson, W. and Maclagan, N.F. The purification and properties of insulin. *Biochem.J.* 21:560-571, 1927.
91. Dische, F.E., Wernstedt, C., Westermark, G.T., Westermark, P., Pepys, M.B., Rennie, J.A., Gilbey, S.G. and Watkins, P.J. Insulin as an amyloid-fibril protein at sites of repeated insulin injections in a diabetic patient. *Diabetologia* 31:158-161, 1988.
92. Donato, A.,Di and D'Alessio, G. Heterogeneity of bovine seminal ribonuclease. *Biochemistry* 20:7232-7237, 1981.
93. Donato, A.,Di, Galletti, P. and D'Alessio, G. Selective deamidation and enzymatic methylation of seminal ribonuclease. *Biochemistry* 25:8361-8368, 1986.

94. Drennan, F.M. The presence of the internal secretion of the pancreas in the blood. *Am.J.Physiol.* 28:396-402, 1911.
95. Dudley, H.W. The purification of insulin and some of its properties. *Biochem.J.* 17:376-390, 1923.
96. Easter, B.R.D., Sutton, D.A. and Drewes, S.E. Crystalline [A21-desamido] bovine insulin. *Hoppe-Seyler's Z.Physiol.Chem.* 359:1229-1236, 1978.
97. Ehrlich, J. and Ratner, I.M. Amyloidosis of the islets of Langerhans. *Amer.J.Pathol.* 38:49-59, 1961.
98. Eichner, H.L., Selam, J.-L., Woertz, L.L., Cornblath, M. and Charles, M.A. Improved metabolic control of diabetes with reduction of occlusions during continuous subcutaneous insulin infusion. *Diab.Nutr.Metab.* 1:283-287, 1988.
99. Ellis, M.M. and Newton, E.B. Changes in the physiological action of insulin induced by exposures to ultraviolet light. *Am.J.Physiol.* 73:530-538, 1925.
100. Emdin, S.O., Dodson, G.G., Cutfield, J.M. and Cutfield, S.M. Role of zinc in insulin biosynthesis. Some possible zinc-insulin interactions in the pancreatic B-cell. *Diabetologia* 19:174-182, 1980.
101. Epstein, A.A. The action of pepsin on insulin. *Proc.Soc.Exp.Biol.Med.* 22:9-11, 1924.
102. Epstein, A.A. and Rosenthal, N. Studies on the relation of the external to the internal secretion of the pancreas I. Biochemical study on the nature of the action of trypsin on insulin. *Am.J.Physiol.* 70:225-239, 1924.
103. Epstein, A.A. and Rosenthal, N. Studies on the relation of the external to the internal secretion of the pancreas II. The effect of trypsin on insulin and its bearing on the causation of diabetes. *Am.J.Physiol.* 71:316-338, 1925.
104. Ernst, M.L. and Schmir, G.L. Isoimides. A kinetic study of the reactions of nucleophiles with N-phenylphthalisoimide. *J.Am.Chem.Soc.* 88:5001-5009, 1966.
105. Fankhauser, S. Neuere Aspekte der Insulintherapie. *Schweiz Med.Wochenschr.* 99:414-420, 1969.
106. Farrant, J.L. and Mercer, E.H. Electron microscopical observations of fibrous insulin. *Biochim.Biophys.Acta* 8:355-359, 1952.
107. Fava, A., Iliceto, A. and Camera, E. Kinetics of the thiol-disulfide exchange. *J.Am.Chem.Soc.* 79:833-838, 1957.
108. Feingold, V., Jenkins, A.B. and Kraegen, E.W. Effect of contact material on vibration-induced insulin aggregation. *Diabetologia* 27:373-378, 1984.
109. Felix, K. and Waldschmidt-Leitz, E. Zur chemischen Natur des Insulins. *Berichte der Deutschen Chemische Gesellschaft* 59:2367-2370, 1926.
110. Fineberg, N.S., Fineberg, S.E., Mahler, R.J. and Linarelli, L.G. Is regular human insulin less immunogenic than repository? *Diabetes* 35 (Suppl.1):91, 1986.(Abstract)
111. Fiore, C. and Dose, K. Biologisch-chemische Wirkungen von ultraviolettem Licht auf Insulin. *Biophysik* 2:340-346, 1965.
112. Fischell, R.E., Radford, W.E. and Saudek, C.D. A programmable implantable medication system: application to diabetes. In: *Proceedings of the 16th Hawaii International Conference on System Science*, Western Periodicals Co., 1983, p. 229-234.
113. Fisher, B.V. and Porter, P.B. Stability of bovine insulin. *J.Pharm.Pharmacol.* 33:203-206, 1981.
114. Flatmark, T. On the heterogeneity of beef heart Cytochrome C. III. A kinetic study of the non-enzymic deamidation of the main subfractions (Cy I–Cy III). *Acta Chem.Scand.* 20:1487-1496, 1966.
115. Florence, T.M. Degradation of protein disulphide bonds in dilute alkali. *Biochem.J.* 189:507-520, 1980.
116. Fojtík, A. and Kopoldová, J. Radiolysis of aqueous solutions of insulin. *Collection Czechoslov.Chem.Commun.* 41:2151-2158, 1976.
117. Foster, G.E., Macdonald, J. and Smart, J.V. The assay of insulin in vitro by fibril formation and precipitation. *J.Pharm.Pharmacol.* 3:897-904, 1951.
118. Freudenberg, K., Dirscherl, W. and Eyer, H. Beitrage zur Chemie des Insulins. 8. Mitteilung über Insulin. *Hoppe-Seyler's Z.Physiol.Chem.* 202:128-158, 1931.
119. Freudenberg, K. and Eyer, H. Beiträge zur Chemie des Insulins. 11. Mitteilung über Insulin. *Hoppe-Seyler's Z.Physiol.Chem.* 213:226-247, 1932.
120. Freudenberg, K. and Wegmann, T. Der Schwefel des Insulins. 13.Mitteilung über Insulin. *Hoppe-Seyler's Z.Physiol.Chem.* 233:159-171, 1935.

121. Geiger, T. and Clarke, S. Deamidation, isomerization, and racemization at asparaginyl and aspartyl residues in peptides. Succinimide-linked reactions that contribute to protein degradation. *J.Biol.Chem.* 262:785-794, 1987.
122. Gekko, K. and Timasheff, S.N. Mechanism of protein stabilization by glycerol: Preferential hydration in glycerol-water mixtures. *Biochemistry* 20:4667-4676, 1981.
123. Gekko, K. and Timasheff, S.N. Thermodynamic and kinetic examination of protein stabilization by glycerol. *Biochemistry* 20:4677-4686, 1981.
124. Gerlough, T.D. and Bates, R.W. The purification and some properties of insulin. *J.Pharmacol.Exp.Ther.* 45:19-51, 1932.
125. Glenner, G.G., Eanes, E.D., Bladen, H.A., Linke, R.P. and Termine, J.D. β-Pleated sheet fibrils. A comparison of native amyloid with synthetic protein fibrils. *J.Histochem.Cytochem.* 22:1141-1158, 1974.
126. Grau, U., Seipke, G., Obermeier, R. and Thurow, H. Stabile Insulinlösungen für automatische Dosiergeräte. In: *Neue Insuline. 1. Internationales Symposium*, edited by Petersen, K.-G., Schlüter, K.J. and Kerp, L. Freiburg: Freiburg Graphischer Betriebe, 1982, p. 411-419.
127. Grau, U. Chemical stability of insulin in a delivery system environment. *Diabetologia* 28:458-463, 1985.
128. Grau, U. and Saudek, C.D. Stable insulin preparations for implanted insulin pumps. Laboratory and animal trials. *Diabetes* 36:1453-1459, 1987.
129. Grau, U., Geisen, K. and Jährling, P. Preclinical evaluation of a remote-controlled implantable pump with a compatible insulin preparation: Studies on long-term stability of the insulin. *Diab.Nutr.Metab.* 2:43-52, 1989.
130. Gray, W.R. Sequence analysis with dansyl chloride. *Methods Enzymol.* 25:333-344, 1972.
131. Gregory, R., Edwards, S. and Yateman, N.A. Demonstration of insulin transformation products in insulin vials by high-performance liquid chromatography. *Diabetes Care* 14:42-48, 1991.
132. Grodsky, G.M. An assay of insulin by fibril formation from small samples of pancreas. *Biochem.J.* 68:142-145, 1958.
133. Gros, C.L and Labouesse, B. Study of the dansylation reaction of amino acids, peptides and proteins. *European J.Biochem.* 7:463-470, 1969.
134. Hallas-Møller, K. The 'Lente' insulins. *Diabetes* 5:7-14, 1956.
135. Hangauer, D.G., Monzingo, A.F. and Matthews, B.W. An interactive computer graphics study of thermolysin-catalyzed peptide cleavage and inhibition by N-carboxymethyl dipeptides. *Biochemistry* 23:5730-5741, 1984.
136. Hansen, J.F. The self-association of zinc-free human insulin and insulin analogue B13-glutamine. *Biophys.Chem.* 39:107-110, 1991.
137. Hansen, P.E., Brange, J. and Havelund, S. Stabilized insulin preparations and a process for preparation thereof, *US patent* 4,614,730, 1986.
138. Harris, M.D., Davidson, M.B. and Rosenberg, C.S. Simple solution to problem of biostator-induced insulin aggregation. *Diabetes Care* 9:356-358, 1986.
139. Harteneck, A. and Schuler, W. Die Einwirkung von Pepsin und Trypsin-Kinase auf Insulin. *Hoppe-Seyler's Z.Physiol.Chem.* 172:289-299, 1927.
140. Heding, L.G., Larsen, U.D., Markussen, J., Jørgensen, K.H. and Hallund, O. Radioimmumoassays for human, pork and ox C-peptides and related substances. *Horm.Metab.Res.(Suppl.Ser.)* 5:40-44, 1974.
141. Hefford, M.A., Oda, G. and Kaplan, H. Structure-function relationships in the free insulin monomer. *Biochem.J.* 237:663-668, 1986.
142. Helbig, H.-J. *Insulindimere aus der b-Komponente von Insulinpräparationen*, Aachen, Germany: Rheinisch-Westfälische Technische Hochschule (dissertation), 1976.
143. Helmerhorst, E. and Stokes, G.B. Generation of acid-stable and protein-bound persulfide-like residues in alkali- or sulfhydryl-treated insulin by a mechanism consonant with the β-elimination hypothesis of disulfide bond lysis. *Biochemistry* 22:69-75, 1983.
144. Higuchi, T., Eberson, L. and Herd, A.K. The intramolecular facilitated hydrolytic rates of methyl-substituted succinanilic acids. *J.Am.Chem.Soc.* 88:3805-3808, 1966.
145. Hoed, D.,den, Jongh, S.E.,de and Peek, A.E.J. Über das Verhalten von Insulin gegenüber Röntgen-, Radium- und ultravioletten Strahlen. *Biochem.Z.* 205:144-153, 1929.
146. Howell, S.L., Tyhurst, M., Duvefelt, H., Andersson, A. and Hellerström, C. Role of zinc and calcium in the formation and storage of insulin in the pancreatic B-cell. *Cell Tissue Res.* 188:107-118, 1978.

147. Hutchison, K.G. Assessment of gelling in insulin solutions for infusion pumps. *J.Pharm. Pharmacol.* 37:528-531, 1985.
148. Irsigler, K. and Kritz, H. Long-term continuous intravenous insulin therapy with a portable insulin dosage-regulating apparatus. *Diabetes* 28:196-203, 1979.
149. Irsigler, K., Kritz, H., Hagmüller, G., Franetzki, M., Prestele, K., Thurow, H. and Geisen, K. Long-term continuous intraperitoneal insulin infusion with an implanted remote-controlled insulin infusion device. *Diabetes* 30:1072-1075, 1981.
150. Jackman, W.S., Lougheed, W., Marliss, E.B., Zinman, B. and Albisser, A.M. For insulin infusion: a miniature precision peristaltic pump and silicone rubber reservoir. *Diabetes Care* 21:554-557, 1980.
151. Jackson, R.L., Storvick, W.O., Hollinden, C.S., Stroeh, L.E. and Stilz, J.G. Neutral regular insulin. *Diabetes* 21:235-245, 1972.
152. Jacobsen, H., Demandt, A., Moody, A.J. and Sundby, F. Sequence analysis of porcine gut GLI-1. *Biochim.Biophys.Acta* 493:452-459, 1977.
153. James, D.E., Jenkins, A.B., Kraegen, E.W. and Chisholm, D.J. Insulin precipitation in artificial infusion devices. *Diabetologia* 21:554-557, 1981.
154. Jeffrey, P.D. Polymerization behaviour of bovine zinc-insulin at neutral pH. Molecular weight of the subunit and the effect of glucose. *Biochemistry* 13:4441-4447, 1974.
155. Jensen, E.V. Sulfhydryl-disulfide interchange. *Science* 130:1319-1323, 1959.
156. Jensen, H. and Lawder, A. Beiträge zur Chemie des Insulins. XII. Mitteilung über krystallisiertes Insulin. *Hoppe-Seyler's Z.Physiol.Chem.* 190:262-272, 1930.
157. Jensen, H. and Evans, E.A.,Jr. Die Einwirkung von Säure und Alkali auf Insulin. XV. Mitteilung über krystallisiertes Insulin. *Hoppe-Seyler's Z.Physiol.Chem.* 209:134-144, 1932.
158. Jensen, H., Schock, E. and Sollers, E. Studies on crystalline insulin. XVI. The action of ammonium hydroxide and of iodine on insulin. *J.Biol.Chem.* 98:93-99, 1932.
159. Jensen, H., Evans, E.A.,Jr., Pennington, W.D. and Schock, E.D. The action of various reagents on insulin. *J.Biol.Chem.* 114:199-208, 1936.
160. Jensen, H.F. Preparation of insulin. In: *Insulin. Its chemistry and physiology*, New York: The Commonwealth Fund, 1938, p. 22-37.
161. Jensen, H. The chemical study of insulin. *Science* 75:614-618, 1954.
162. Johnson, B.A., Shirokawa, J.M., Hancock, W.S., Spellman, M.W., Basa, L.J. and Aswad, D.W. Formation of isoaspartate at two distinct sites during in vitro ageing of human growth hormone. *J.Biol.Chem.* 264:14262-14271, 1989.
163. Johnson, K.H. and Stevens, J.B. Light and electron microscopic studies of islet amyloid in diabetic cats. *Diabetes* 22:81-90, 1972.
164. Jollès, P. and Fromageot, C. Caractérisation du résidu β-aspartique (–NH·CH(COOH)CH2·CO–) dans l'insuline. *Biochim.Biophys.Acta* 9:416-418, 1952.
165. Jones, A.J., Helmerhorst, E. and Stokes, G.B. The formation of dehydroalanine residues in alkali-treated insulin and oxidized glutathione. *Biochem.J.* 211:499-502, 1983.
166. Jorpes, J.E. Recrystallized insulin for diabetic patients with insulin allergy. *Arch.Intern.Med.* 833:363-371, 1949.
167. Jørgensen, K.H., Brange, J., Hallund, O. and Pingel, M. A method for the preparation of essentially pure insulin. In: *VII. Congress of the International Diabetes Federation* (International Congress Series No. 209), edited by Rodrigues, R.R., Ebling, F.J.G., Henderson, I. and Assan, R. Amsterdam: Excerpta Medica Foundation, 1970, p. 149.
168. Jørgensen, K.H. and Larsen, U.D. Homogeneous mono-125I-insulins. Preparation and characterization of mono-125I-(Tyr A14)- and mono-125I-(Tyr A19)-insulin. *Diabetologia* 19:546-554, 1980.
169. Kaplan, E.H., Campbell, E.D. and McLaren, A.D. Photochemistry of proteins. VIII. Inactivation of insulin by ultraviolet light. *Biochim.Biophys.Acta* 4:493-500, 1950.
170. Katsoyannis, P.G. The synthesis of the insulin chains and their combination to biologically active material. *Diabetes* 13:339-348, 1964.
171. Kedar, I., Ravid, M. and Sohar, E. In vitro synthesis of "amyloid" fibrils from insulin, calcitonin and parathormone. *Isr.J.Med.Sci.* 12:1137-1140, 1976.
172. Kirby, A.J. and Lancaster, P.W. Structure and efficiency in intramolecular and enzymic catalysis. Catalysis of amide hydrolysis by the carboxy- group of substituted maleamic acids. *J.Chem.Soc.Perkin Trans.* 2:1206-1214, 1972.

173. Kirby, A.J. Effective molarities for intramolecular reactions. In: *Advances in physical organic chemistry* vol. 17, edited by Gold, V. and Bethell, D. London, New York: Academic Press, 1980, p. 183-278.
174. Kirk, K.L. and Cohen, L.A. Intramolecular aminolysis of amides. Effects of electronic variations in the attacking and leaving groups. *J.Am.Chem.Soc.* 94:8142-8147, 1972.
175. Kluger, R. and Lam, C.-H. Rate-determining processes in the hydrolysis of maleanilinic acids in acidic solutions. *J.Am.Chem.Soc.* 98:4154-4158, 1976.
176. Kluger, R. and Lam, C.-H. Carboxylic acid participation in amide hydrolysis. External general base and general acid catalysis in reactions of norbornenylanilic acids. *J.Am.Chem.Soc.* 100:2191-2197, 1978.
177. Knowlton, F.P. and Starling, E.H. Experiments on the consumption of sugar in the normal and the diabetic heart. *J.Physiol.* 45:146-163, 1912.
178. Koltun, W.L., Waugh, D.F. and Bear, R.S. An x-ray diffraction investigation of selected types of insulin fibrils. *J.Am.Chem.Soc.* 76:413-417, 1954.
179. Kopoldová, J. Radiation aggregates of insulin. *Z.Naturforsch.* 34c:1139-1143, 1979.
180. Kossiakoff, A.A. Tertiary structure is a principal determinant to protein deamidation. *Science* 240:191-194, 1988.
181. Krayenbühl, C. and Rosenberg, T. Crystalline protamine insulin. *Rep.Steno Mem.Hosp.Nord. Insulinlab.* 1:60-73, 1946.
182. Krogh, A. and Hemmingsen, A.M. The destructive action of heat on insulin solutions. *Biochem. J.* 22:1231-1238, 1928.
183. Kuhn, W., Eyer, H. and Freudenberg, K. Das optische Verhalten des Insulins und seiner Derivate. 6. Mitteilung über Insulin. *Hoppe-Seyler's Z.Physiol.Chem.* 202:97-115, 1931.
184. Kung, T.H. and Tsao, T.C. The ultrastructure of insulin fibrils. *Sci.Sin.* 13:471-478, 1964.
185. Kung, Y.-T., Du, Y.-C., Huang, W.-T., Chen, C.-C., Ke, L.-T., Hu, S.-C., Jiang, R.-Q., Chu, S.-Q., Niu, C.-I., Hsu, J.-Z., Chang, W.-C, Chen, L.-L., Li, H.-S., Wang, Y., Loh, T.-P., Chi, A.-H., Li, C.-H., Shi, P.-T., Yieh, Y.-H., Tang, K.-L. and Hsing, C.-Y. The total synthesis of crystalline insulin. *Sci.Sinica* 15:544-561, 1966.
186. Küstner, H. and Eissner, W. Beeinflussung des Insulins durch rote und ultraviolette Bestrahlung. *Klin.Wochenschr.* 11:499-501, 1932.
187. Küstner, H. and Eissner, W. Über den Einfluss von ultraviolettem Licht auf die physiologische Wirksamkeit des Insulins. *Klin.Wochenschr.* 11:1668-1669, 1932.
188. Langmuir, I. and Waugh, D.F. Pressure-soluble and pressure-displaceable components of monolayers of native and denatured proteins. *J.Am.Chem.Soc.* 62:2771-2793, 1940.
189. Leach, S.J. and Lindley, H. The kinetics of hydrolysis of the amide group in proteins and peptides. Part 1. The acid hydrolysis of l-asparagine and l-asparaginylglycine. *Trans.Faraday Soc.* 49:915-920, 1953.
190. Leach, S.J. and Lindley, H. The kinetics of hydrolysis of the amide group in proteins and peptides. Part 2. Acid hydrolysis of glycyl- and l-leucyl-l-asparagine. *Trans.Faraday Soc.* 49:921-925, 1953.
191. Lee, L.L.-Y. and Lee, J.C. Thermal stability of proteins in the presence of poly(ethylene glycols). *Biochemistry* 26:7813-7819, 1987.
192. Lens, J. The inactivation of insulin solutions. *J.Biol.Chem.* 169:313-322, 1947.
193. Lens, J. The preparation and properties of pure insulin. *Biochim.Biophys.Acta* 2:76-79, 1948.
194. Light, A. and Simpson, M.V. Studies on the biosynthesis of insulin. I. The paper chromatographic isolation of 14C-labeled insulin from calf pancreas slices. *Biochim.Biophys.Acta* 20:251-261, 1956.
195. Light, A. Leucine aminopeptidase in sequence determination of peptides. *Methods Enzymol.* 25:253-262, 1972.
196. Lou, S., Liao, C., McClelland, J.F. and Graves, D.J. Formation of a cyclic imide in aspartyl or asparaginyl glycyl peptides induced by heating in the dry state. *Int.J.Peptide Protein Res.* 29:728-733, 1987.
197. Lougheed, W.D., Woulfe-Flanagan, H., Clement, J.R. and Albisser, A.M. Insulin aggregation in artificial delivery systems. *Diabetologia* 19:1-9, 1980.
198. Lougheed, W.D., Albisser, A.M., Martindale, H.M., Chow, J.C. and Clement, J.R. Physical stability of insulin formulations. *Diabetes* 32:424-432, 1983.
199. Lura, R. and Schirch, V. Role of peptide conformation in the rate and mechanism of deamidation of asparaginyl residues. *Biochemistry* 27:7671-7677, 1988.

200. Macleod, J.J.R. *Insulin. Its use in the treatment of diabetes*, Baltimore:Williams & Wilkins, 1925.
201. Maislos, M., Mead, P.M., Gaynor, D.H. and Robbins, D.C. The source of the circulating aggregate of insulin in type I diabetic patients is therapeutic insulin. *J.Clin.Invest.* 77:717-723, 1986.
202. Manning, M.C., Patel, K. and Borchardt, R.T. Stability of protein pharmaceuticals. *Pharm.Res.* 6:903-918, 1989.
203. Markussen, J., Diers, I., Hougaard, P., Langkjaer, L., Norris, K., Snel, L., Sørensen, A.R., Sørensen, E. and Voigt, H.O. Soluble, prolonged-acting insulin derivatives. III. Degree of protraction, crystallizability and chemical stability of insulins substituted in position A21, B13, B23, B27 and B30. *Protein Eng.* 2:157-166, 1988.
204. McFadden, P.N. and Clarke, S. Conversion of isoaspartyl peptides to normal peptides: Implications for the cellular repair of damaged proteins. *Proc.Natl.Acad.Sci.USA* 84:2595-2599, 1987.
205. McGraw, S.E., Craik, D.J. and Lindenbaum, S. Testing of insulin hexamer-stabilizing ligands using theoretical binding, microcalorimetry, and nuclear magnetic resonance (NMR) line broadening techniques. *Pharm.Res.* 7:600-605, 1990.
206. McGraw, S.E. and Lindenbaum, S. The use of microcalorimetry to measure thermodynamic parameters of the binding of ligands to insulin. *Pharm.Res.* 7:606-611, 1990.
207. McKerrow, J.H. and Robinson, A.B. Deamidation of asparaginyl residues as a hazard in experimental protein and peptide procedures. *Anal.Biochem.* 42:565-568, 1971.
208. Mecklenburg, R.S. and Guinn, T.S. Complications of insulin pump therapy: The effect of insulin preparation. *Diabetes Care* 8:367-370, 1985.
209. Meienhofer, J., Schnabel, E., Bremer, H., Brinkhoff, O., Zabel, R., Sroka, W., Klostermeyer, H., Brandenburg, D., Okuda, T. and Zahn, H. Synthese der Insulinketten und ihre Kombination zu insulinaktiven Präparaten. *Z.Naturforsch.* 18B:1120-1121, 1963.
210. Meinwald, Y.C., Stimson, E.R. and Scheraga, H.A. Deamidation of the asparaginyl-glycyl sequence. *Int.J.Peptide Protein Res.* 28:79-84, 1986.
211. Melberg, S.G., Havelund, S., Villumsen, J. and Brange, J. Insulin compatibility with polymer materials used in external pump infusion systems. *Diabetic Med.* 5:243-247, 1988.
212. Mering, J.,von and Minkowski, O. Diabetes mellitus nach Pankreasextirpation. *Arch.f.exper. Path.u.Pharmakol.* 26:371-387, 1890.
213. Miller, H.K. and Waelsch, H. Utilization of glutamine and asparagine and their peptides by micro-organisms. *Nature* 169:30-31, 1952.
214. Milstien, S. and Cohen, L.A. Stereopopulation control. I. Rate enhancement in the lactonizations of o-hydroxyhydrocinnamic acids. *J.Am.Chem.Soc.* 94:9158-9165, 1972.
215. Mirsky, I.A. and Kawamura, K. Heterogeneity of crystalline insulin. *Endocrinology* 78:1115-1119, 1966.
216. Mommaerts, W.F.H.M. and Neurath, H. Insulin methyl ester. I. Preparation and properties. *J.Biol.Chem.* 185:909-917, 1950.
217. Moody, A.J., Thim, L. and Valverde, I. The isolation and sequencing of human gastric inhibitory peptide (GIP). *Febs Lett.* 172:142-148, 1984.
218. Murlin, J.R., Clough, H.D., Gibbs, C.B.F. and Stokes, A.M. Aqueous extracts of pancreas I. Influence on the carbohydrate metabolism of depancreatized animals. *J.Biol.Chem.* 56:253-296, 1923.
219. Nagasawa, K., Nakayama, G., Serizawa, J., Sato, H. and Shirai, J. Studies on the sterilization of hormone preparations through radiation of 60Co. *Bulletin of the National Institute of Hygienic Sciences* 75:5-6, 1957.
220. Nashef, A.S., Osuga, D.T., Lee, H.S., Ahmed, A.I., Whitaker, J.R. and Feeney, R.E. Effects of alkali on proteins. Disulfides and their products. *J.Agric.Food Chem.* 25:245-251, 1977.
221. Nell, L.J. and Thomas, J.W. Frequency and specificity of protamine antibodies in diabetic and control subjects. *Diabetes* 37:172-176, 1988.
222. Nunes-Correa, J., Lowy, C. and Sönksen, P.H. Presumed insulinoma secreting a high-molecular-weight insulin analogue. *Lancet* 1:837-841, 1974.
223. Ota, I.M. and Clarke, S. Enzymatic methylation of l-isoaspartyl residues derived from aspartyl residues in affinity-purified calmodulin. The role of conformational flexibility in spontaneous isoaspartyl formation. *J.Biol.Chem.* 264:54-60, 1989.
224. Ota, I.M. and Clarke, S. Calcium affects the spontaneous degradation of aspartyl/asparaginyl residues in calmodulin. *Biochemistry* 28:4020-4027, 1989.

225. Palmieri, R., Lee, R.W.-K. and Dunn, M.F. 1H Fourier transform NMR studies of insulin: Coordination of Ca^{2+} to the Glu(B13) site drives hexamer assembly and induces a conformation change. *Biochemistry* 27:3387-3397, 1988.

226. Patel, K. and Borchardt, R.T. Chemical pathways of peptide degradation. II. Kinetics of deamidation of an asparaginyl residue in a model hexapeptide. *Pharm.Res.* 7:703-711, 1990.

227. Patel, K. and Borchardt, R.T. Chemical pathways of peptide degradation. III. Effect of primary sequence on the pathways of deamidation of asparaginyl residues in hexapeptides. *Pharm.Res.* 7:787-793, 1990.

228. Perry, E.K., Oakley, A.E., Candy, J.M. and Perry, R.H. Properties and possible significance of substance P and insulin fibrils. *Neurosci. Lett.* 25:321-325, 1981.

229. Pettinga, C.W. Insulin. *Biochemical Preparations* 6:28-31, 1958.

230. Phillips, D.M.P. and Mercer, E.H. Fibrous insulin (F-insulin). *Biochim.Biophys.Acta* 12:592-593, 1953.

231. Pickup, J.C., Keen, H., Parsons, A.J. and Alberti, K.G.M.M. Continuous subcutaneous insulin infusion: An approach to achieving normoglycaemia. *Br.Med.J.* 1:204-207, 1978.

232. Pietri, A. and Raskin, P. Cutaneous complications of chronic continuous subcutaneous insulin infusion therapy. *Diabetes Care* 4:624-626, 1981.

233. Pingel, M. and Vølund, A. Stability of insulin preparations. *Diabetes* 21:805-813, 1972.

234. Pongor, S., Brownlee, M. and Cerami, A. Preparation of high-potency, non-aggregating insulins using a novel sulfation procedure. *Diabetes* 32:1087-1091, 1983.

235. Porter, R.R. The reactivity of the iminazole ring in proteins. *Biochem.J.* 46:304-307, 1950.

236. Prestele, K., Franetzki, M. and Kresse, H. Development of program-controlled portable insulin delivery device. *Diabetes Care* 3:362-368, 1980.

237. Quinn, R. and Andrade, J.D. Minimizing the aggregation of neutral insulin solutions. *J.Pharm.Sci.* 72:1472-1473, 1983.

238. Rasch, R. Control of blood glucose levels in the streptozotocin diabetic rat using a long-acting heat-treated insulin. *Diabetologia* 16:185-190, 1979.

239. Ratner, R.E. and Steiner, M.L. Insulin-pump therapy: Effect of phosphate-buffered human insulin. *Diabetes Care* 10:787-788, 1987.

240. Ratner, R.E., Phillips, T.M. and Steiner, M. Persistent cutaneous insulin allergy resulting from high-molecular-weight insulin aggregates. *Diabetes* 39:728-733, 1990.

241. Reeves, W.G. Immunogenicity of insulin of various origins. *Neth.J.Med.* 28 (Suppl.1):43-46, 1985.

242. Reinscheidt, H., Strassburger, W., Glatter, U., Wollmer, A., Dodson, G.G. and Mercola, D.A. A solution equivalent of the 2Zn→4Zn transformation of insulin in the crystal. *Eur.J.Biochem.* 142:7-14, 1984.

243. Reisfeld, R.A., Lewis, U.J. and Williams, D.E. Disk electrophoresis of basic proteins and peptides on polyacrylamide gels. *Nature* 195:281-283, 1962.

244. Rice, E.W. The preparation of formazin standards for nephelometry. *Anal.Chim.Acta* 87:251-253, 1976.

245. Robbins, D.C., Cooper, S.M., Fineberg, S.E. and Mead, P.M. Antibodies to covalent aggregates of insulin in blood of insulin-using diabetic patients. *Diabetes* 36:838-841, 1987.

246. Robbins, D.C. and Mead, P.M. Free covalent aggregates of therapeutic insulin in the blood of insulin-dependent diabetics. *Diabetes* 36:147-151, 1987.

247. Robinson, A.B. and Rudd, C.J. Deamidation of glutaminyl and asparaginyl residues in peptides and proteins. In: *Current Topics in Cellular Regulation*, Vol. 8, edited by Horecker, B.L. and Stadtman, E.R. New York: Academic Press, 1974, p. 247-295.

248. Roy, M., Lee, R.W.K., Brange, J. and Dunn, M.F. 1H NMR spectrum of the native human insulin monomer: Evidence for conformational differences between the monomer and aggregated forms. *J.Biol.Chem.* 265:5448-5452, 1990.

249. Ryle, A.P. and Sanger, F. Disulphide interchange reactions. *Biochem.J.* 60:535-540, 1955.

250. Ryle, A.P., Sanger, F. and Kitai, R. The disulphide bonds of insulin. *Biochem.J.* 60:541-556, 1955.

251. Sahyun, M., Goodell, M. and Nixon, A. Factors influencing the stability of insulin. *J.Biol.Chem.* 117:685-691, 1937.

252. Sahyun, M., Nixon, A. and Goodell, M. Influence of certain metals on the stability of insulin. *J.Pharmacol.Exp.Ther.* 65:143-149, 1939.

253. Sanger, F., Thompson, E.O.P. and Kitai, R. The amide groups of insulin. *Biochem.J.* 59:509-518, 1955.
254. Sato, T., Ebert, C.D. and Kim, S.W. Prevention of insulin self-association and surface adsorption. *J.Pharm.Sci.* 72:228-232, 1983.
255. Sauers, C.K., Marikakis, C.A. and Lupton, M.A. Synthesis of saturated isoimides. Reactions of N-phenyl- 2,2-dimethylsuccinisoimide with aqueous buffer solutions. *J.Am.Chem.Soc.* 95:6792-6799, 1973.
256. Schade, D.S., Eaton, R.P., DeLongo, J., Saland, L.C., Ladman, A.J. and Carlson, G.A. Electron microscopy of insulin precipitates. *Diabetes Care* 5:25-30, 1982.
257. Schade, D.S., Eaton, R.P., Edwards, S., Doberneck, R.C., Spencer, W.J., Carlson, G.A.B, Bair, R.E., Love, J.T., Urenda, R.S. and Gaona, J.I.,Jr. A remotely programmable insulin delivery system. Successful short-term implantation in man. *JAMA* 247:1848-1853, 1982.
258. Schlichtkrull, J. *Insulin crystals. Chemical and biological studies on insulin crystals and insulin zinc suspensions,* (Thesis), Copenhagen:Munksgaard Publisher, 1958.
259. Schlichtkrull, J., Funder, J. and Munck, O. Clinical evaluation of a new insulin preparation. In: *4e Congrès de la Féderation Internationale du Diabète,* Genève, edited by Demole, M. Genève: Editions Médecine et Hygiène, 1961, p. 303-305.
260. Schlichtkrull, J., Munck, O. and Jersild, M. Insulin Rapitard and insulin Actrapid. *Acta Med.Scand.* 177:103-113, 1965.
261. Schlichtkrull, J., Brange, J., Christiansen, A.H., Hallund, O., Heding, L.G. and Jørgensen, K.H. Clinical aspects of insulin – antigenicity. *Diabetes* 21 (suppl. 2):649-656, 1972.
262. Schlichtkrull, J., Brange, J., Christiansen, A.H., Hallund, O., Heding, L.G., Jørgensen, K.H., Rasmussen, S.M., Sørensen, E. and Vølund, A. Monocomponent insulin and its clinical implications. *Horm.Metab.Res. (Suppl.Ser.)* 5:134-143, 1974.
263. Schlichtkrull, J., Pingel, M., Heding, L.G., Brange, J. and Jørgensen, K.H. Insulin preparations with prolonged effect. In: *Handbook of Experimental Pharmacology, New Series,* vol XXXII/2, edited by Hasselblatt, A. and Bruchhausen, F. Berlin, Heidelberg, New York: Springer-Verlag, 1975, p. 729-777.
264. Schneider, H.-M., Störkel, F.S. and Will, W. The influence of insulin on local amyloidosis of the islets of Langerhans and insulinoma. *Path.Res.Pract.* 170:180-191, 1980.
265. Scotchler, J.W. and Robinson, A.B. Deamidation of glutaminyl residues: Dependence on pH, temperature, and ionic strength. *Anal.Biochem.* 59:319-322, 1974.
266. Scott, D.A. The action of trypsin on insulin. *J.Biol.Chem.* 63:641-651, 1925.
267. Scott, D.A. A further investigation of the chemical properties of insulin. *J.Biol.Chem.* 65:601-616, 1925.
268. Scott, D.A. Crystalline insulin. *Biochem.J.* 28:1592-1602, 1934.
269. Scott, E.L. On the influence of intravenous injections of an extract of the pancreas on experimental pancreatic diabetes. *Am.J.Physiol.* 29:306-310, 1911.
270. Seiler, N. and Wiechmann, J. Zum Nachweis von Aminosäuren im 10^{-10}-Mol-Masstab. Trennung von 1-Dimethylamino-naphthalin-5-sulfonyl-aminosäuren auf Dünnschicht-chromatogrammen. *Experientia* 20/10:559-560, 1964.
271. Selam, J.-L., Zirinis, P., Mellet, M. and Mirouze, J. Stable insulin for implantable delivery systems: In vitro studies with different containers and solvents. *Diabetes Care* 10:343-347, 1987.
272. Sestoft, L., Vølund, A., Gammeltoft, S., Birch, K. and Hildebrandt, P. The biological properties of human insulin. *Acta Med.Scand.* 212:21-28, 1982.
273. Shalitin, Y. and Bernhard, S.A. Neighboring effects on ester hydrolysis. I. Neighboring hydroxyl groups. *J.Am.Chem.Soc.* 86:2291-2292, 1964.
274. Shalitin, Y. and Bernhard, S.A. Cooperative effects of functional groups in peptides. II. Elimination reactions in aspartyl-(O-acyl)-serine derivatives. *J.Am.Chem.Soc.* 88:4711-4721, 1966.
275. Shifrin, S. and Parrott, C.L. Influence of glycerol and other polyhydric alcohols on the quaternary structure of an oligomeric protein. *Arch.Biochem.Biophys.* 166:426-432, 1975.
276. Shonle, H.A. and Waldo, J.H. Some chemical reactions of the substance containing insulin. *J.Biol.Chem.* 58:731-736, 1923.
277. Shonle, H.A. and Waldo, J.H. The destructive action of acids, alkalies, and enzymes on insulin. *J.Biol.Chem.* 66:467-474, 1925.
278. Siebert, W., Fiore, C. and Dose, K. Aminosäureveränderungen in Rinderinsulin durch UV-Bestrahlung. *Z.Naturforschg.* 20b:957-959, 1965.

279. Simkin, R.D., Cole, S.A., Ozawa, H., Magdoff-Fairchild, B., Eggena, P., Rudko, A. and Low, B.W. Precipitation and crystallization of insulin in the presence of lysozyme and salmine. *Biochim.Biophys.Acta* 200:385-394, 1970.

280. Slobin, L.I. and Carpenter, F.H. The labile amide in insulin: Preparation of desalanine- desamido-insulin. *Biochemistry* 2:22-28, 1963.

281. Slobin, L.I. *The action of carboxypeptidase A on bovine insulin and related model peptides,* (Dissertation), Berkeley: University of California, 1964.

282. Sluzky, V., Tamada, J.A., Klibanov, A.M. and Langer, R. Kinetics of insulin aggregation in aqueous solutions upon agitation in the presence of hydrophobic surfaces. *Proc.Natl.Acad. Sci.USA* 88:9377-9381, 1991.

283. Sluzky, V., Klibanov, A.M. and Langer, R. Mechanism of insulin aggregation and stabilization in agitated aqueous solutions. *Biotechnology and Bioengineering* 40:895-903, 1992.

284. Smith, G.D. and Dodson, G.G. Structure of a rhombohedral R6 insulin/phenol complex. *Proteins: Structure, Function, and Genetics* 14:401-408, 1992.

285. Soboleva, N.N., Ivanova, A.I., Talrose, V.L., Trofimov, V.I. and Fedotov, V.P. Radiation resistivity of frozen insulin solutions and suspensions. *International Journal of Applied Radiation and Isotopes* 32:753-756, 1981.

286. Sondheimer, E. and Holley, R.W. Imides from asparagine and glutamine. *J.Am.Chem.Soc.* 76:2467-2470, 1954.

287. Springell, P.H. Reaction of iodine with insulin and fibrous insulin. *Biochim.Biophys.Acta* 63:136-149, 1962.

288. Steiner, D.F. Evidence for a precursor in the biosynthesis of insulin. *Trans.N.Y.Acad.Sci.* 30(Ser.II):60-68, 1967.

289. Steiner, D.F., Hallund, O., Rubenstein, A., Cho, S. and Bayliss, C. Isolation and properties of proinsulin, intermediate forms, and other minor components from crystalline bovine insulin. *Diabetes* 17:725-736, 1968.

290. Steiner, D.F. Proinsulin and the biosynthesis of insulin. *N.Engl.J.Med.* 280:1106-1113, 1969.

291. Stephenson, N.R. and Romans, R.G. Thermal stability of insulin made from zinc insulin crystals. *J.Pharm.Pharmacol.* 12:372-376, 1960.

292. Stephenson, R.C. and Clarke, S. Succinimide formation from aspartyl and asparaginyl peptides as a model for the spontaneous degradation of proteins. *J.Biol.Chem.* 264:6164-6170, 1989.

293. Storvick, W.O. and Henry, H.J. Effect of storage temperature on stability of commercial insulin preparations. *Diabetes* 17:499-502, 1968.

294. Störkel, S., Schneider, H.-M., Müntefering, H. and Kashiwagi, S. Iatrogenic, insulin-dependent, local amyloidosis. *Lab.Invest.* 48:108-111, 1983.

295. Sudmeier, J.L., Bell, S.J., Storm, M.C. and Dunn, M.F. Cadmium-113 nuclear magnetic resonance studies of bovine insulin: Two-zinc hexamer specifically binds calcium. *Science* 212:560-562, 1981.

296. Sundby, F. Separation and characterization of acid-induced insulin transformation products by paper electrophoresis in 7 M urea. *J.Biol.Chem.* 237:3406-3411, 1962.

297. Swanenpoel, O.A., Mellet, P. and Scanes, G. Photolysis of the disulfide linkages in insulin. *Arch.Biochem.Biophys.* 129:26-29, 1969.

298. Tamborlane, W.V., Sherwin, R.S., Genel, M. and Felig, P. Reduction to normal of plasma glucose in juvenile diabetes by subcutaneous administration of insulin with a portable infusion pump. *N.Engl.J.Med.* 300:573-578, 1979.

299. Termine, J.D., Eanes, E.D., Ein, D. and Glenner, G.G. Infrared spectroscopy of human amyloid fibrils and immunoglobulin proteins. *Biopolymers* 11:1103-1113, 1972.

300. Teshima, G., Stults, J.T., Ling, V. and Canova-Davis, E. Isolation and characterization of a succinimide variant of methionyl human growth hormone. *J.Biol.Chem.* 266:13544-13547, 1991.

301. Thurow, H. Studies on the denaturation of dissolved insulin. In: *Insulin. Chemistry, Structure and Function of Insulin and Related Hormones,* edited by Brandenburg, D. and Wollmer, A. Berlin, New York: Gruyter, 1980, p. 215-221.

302. Thurow, H. and Geisen, K. Stabilisation of dissolved proteins against denaturation at hydrophobic interfaces. *Diabetologia* 27:212-218, 1984.

303. Toma, S., Campagnoli, S., Gregoris, E.,De, Gianna, R., Margarit, I., Zamai, M. and Grandi, G. Effect of Glu-143 and His-231 substitutions on the catalytic activity and secretion of bacillus subtilis neutral protease. *Protein Eng.* 2:359-364, 1989.

304. Torchinsky, Y.M. *Sulfur in proteins,* Oxford:Pergamon Press, 1981. p. 1-294.

305. Tsuda, T., Uchiyama, M., Sato, T., Yoshino, H., Tsuchiya, Y., Ishikawa, S., Ohmae, M., Watanabe, S. and Miyake, Y. Mechanism and kinetics of secretin degradation in aqueous solutions. *J.Pharm.Sci.* 79:223-227, 1990.
306. Turnell, W.G. and Finch, J.T. Binding of the dye congo red to the amyloid protein pig insulin reveals a novel homology amongst amyloid-forming peptide sequences. *J.Mol.Biol.* 227:1205-1223, 1992.
307. Tyler-Cross, R. and Schirch, V. Effects of amino acid sequence, buffers, and ionic strength on the rate and mechanism of deamidation of asparagine residues in small peptides. *J.Biol.Chem.* 266:22549-22556, 1991.
308. Vallee, B.L. and Auld, D.S. Zinc coordination, function, and structure of zinc enzymes and other proteins. *Biochemistry* 29:5647-5659, 1990.
309. Varandani, P.T. A convenient preparation of reduced and S-sulfonated A and B chains of insulin. *Biochim.Biophys.Acta* 127:246-249, 1966.
310. Vigneaud, V.,du, Geiling, E.M.K. and Eddy, C.A. Studies on crystalline insulin. VI. Further contributions to the question whether or not crystalline insulin is an adsorption product. *J.Pharmacol.Exp.Ther.* 33:497-509, 1928.
311. Vigneaud, V.,du The "heat precipitate" of crystalline insulin. *J.Biol.Chem.* 92:liv-llv, 1931.
312. Vigneaud, V.,du, Fitch, A., Pekarek, E. and Lockwood, W.W. The inactivation of crystalline insulin by cysteine and gluthathione. *J.Biol.Chem.* 94:233-242, 1931.
313. Vigneaud, V.,du, Sifferd, R.H. and Sealock, R.R. The heat precipitation of insulin. *J.Biol.Chem.* 102:521-533, 1933.
314. Violand, B.N., Schlittler, M.R., Toren, P.C. and Siegel, N.R. Formation of isoaspartate 99 in bovine and porcine somatropins. *J.Protein Chem.* 9:109-117, 1990.
315. Volkin, D.B. and Klibanov, A.M. Thermal destruction processes in proteins involving cystine residues. *J.Biol.Chem.* 262:2945-2950, 1987.
316. Voorter, C.E.M., Haard-Hoekman, W.A.,de, Oetelaar, P.J.M.,van den, Bloemendal, H. and Jong, W.W.,de. Spontaneous peptide bond cleavage in ageing α-crystallin through a succinimide intermediate. *J.Biol.Chem.* 263:19020-19023, 1988.
317. Waugh, D.F. The properties of protein fibers produced reversibly from soluble protein molecules. *Am.J.Physiol.* 133:P484-P485, 1941.
318. Waugh, D.F. The linkage of corpuscular protein molecules. I. A fibrous modification of insulin. *J.Am.Chem.Soc.* 66:663, 1944.
319. Waugh, D.F. A fibrous modification of insulin. I. The heat precipitate of insulin. *J.Am.Chem.Soc.* 68:247-250, 1946.
320. Waugh, D.F. Reactions involved in insulin fibril formation. *Federation Proc.* 5:111, 1946.
321. Waugh, D.F. Regeneration of insulin from insulin fibrils by the action of alkali. *J.Am.Chem.Soc.* 70:1850-1857, 1948.
322. Waugh, D.F., Smith, M.J. and Fearing, D.F. Regeneration of insulin fibrils with several reagents and the nature of the inter-insulin bond. *Federation Proc.* 7:131, 1948.
323. Waugh, D.F., Thompson, R.E. and Weimer, R.J. Assay of insulin in vitro by fibril elongation and precipitation. *J.Biol.Chem.* 185:85-95, 1950.
324. Waugh, D.F., Wilhelmson, D.F., Commerford, S.L. and Sackler, M.L. Studies on the nucleation and growth reactions of selected types of insulin fibrils. *J.Am.Chem.Soc.* 75:2592-2600, 1953.
325. Waugh, D.F. Protein-protein interactions. *Adv.Prot.Chem.* 9:325-437, 1954.
326. Waugh, D.F. A mechanism for the formation of fibrils from protein molecules. *J.Cell.Comp. Physiol.* 49 (Suppl.1):145-164, 1957.
327. Wearne, S.J. and Creighton, T.E. Effect of protein conformation on rate of deamidation: Ribonuclease A. *Proteins: Struct.Funct.Genet.* 5:8-12, 1989.
328. Weiss, S. and Pogány, J. Über die Wirkung der Verdauungsfermente auf das Insulin. *Z.Exp.Med.* 50:786-794, 1926.
329. Westermark, P. On the nature of the amyloid in human islets of Langerhans. *Histochemistry* 38:27-33, 1974.
330. Westermark, P., Grimelius, L., Polak, J.M., Larsson, L.-I., Noorden, S., Wilander, E. and Pearse, A.G.E. Amyloid in polypeptide hormone-producing tumors. *Lab.Invest.* 37:212-215, 1977.
331. Westermark, P. and Wilander, E. Islet amyloid in type 2 (non-insulin-dependent) diabetes is related to insulin. *Diabetologia* 24:342-346, 1983.
332. Wintersteiner, O. The action of sulfhydryl compounds on insulin. *J.Biol.Chem.* 102:473-488, 1933.

333. Witzemann, E.J. and Livshis, L. The action of ammonium hydroxide and other alkaline compounds on insulin. *J.Biol.Chem.* 58:463-474, 1923.
334. Witzemann, E.J. and Livshis, L. The action of proteolytic enzymes upon insulin. *J.Biol.Chem.* 57:425-435, 1923.
335. Wollmer, A., Rannefeld, B., Johansen, B.R., Hejnaes, K.R., Balschmidt, P. and Hansen, F.B. Phenol-promoted structural transformation of insulin in solution. *Biol.Chem.Hoppe-Seyler* 368:903-911, 1987.
336. Wright, H.T. and Robinson, A.B. Cryptic amidase active sites catalyze deamidation in proteins. In: *From cyclotrons to cytochromes. Essays in molecular biology and chemistry*, edited by Kaplan, N.O. and Robinson, A. New York, London: Academic Press, 1982, p. 727-743.
337. Wright, H.T. Sequence and structure determinants of the nonenzymatic deamidation of asparagine and glutamine residues in proteins. *Protein Eng.* 4:283-294, 1991.
338. Wrigley, C. Gel electrofocusing – a technique for analyzing multiple protein samples by isoelectric focusing. *Science Tools* 15:17-23, 1968.
339. Yu, N.T., Jo, B.H., Chang, R.C.C. and Huber, J.D. Single-crystal raman spectra of native insulin. Structures of insulin fibrils, glucagon fibrils, and intact calf lens. *Arch.Biochem.Biophys.* 160:614-622, 1974.
340. Yüksel, K.. and Gracy, R.W. In vitro deamidation of human triosephosphate isomerase. *Arch.Biochem.Biophys.* 248:452-459, 1986.

Formulation of Physically Stable Neutral Insulin Solutions for Continuous Infusion by Delivery Systems

Jens Brange, Svend Havelund, Philip E. Hansen, Lotte Langkjaer, Else Sørensen, and Per Hildebrandt

Novo Research Institute, DK-2880 Bagsvaerd, Denmark, and Hvidore Hospital, DK-2930 Klampenborg, Denmark

Commercial insulin solutions are not sufficiently stable for long-term use in implantable infusion systems. Physical and chemical stability of insulin solutions varies with formulation of the preparations. Furthermore, physical stability has been found to decrease with increasing purity of insulin; this probably explains differences in physical stability between different brands of insulin of similar formulation.

An additive for physical stabilization of insulin must be physiologically acceptable, compatible, and without negative influence on insulin quality. Most additives reported to improve physical stability have been found to impair chemical and biological stability. However, addition of Ca^{++} in low concentrations has been shown to increase physical stability of neutral insulin solutions without affecting the quality of the insulin, including timing and immunological characteristics.

Certain materials used for construction of pump fluid systems increase the tendency of insulin to form insoluble precipitates. Therefore, proper selection and testing of the construction materials are imperative, necessitating close collaboration between insulin and pump manufacturers.

It is concluded that in developing insulin preparations suitable for constant infusion, not only physical but chemical, biological, and immunological properties, as well as material compatibility, must be considered.

The neutral insulin solution introduced as Actrapid nearly 20 years ago (Schlichtkrull, Munck, and Jersild, 1965) can be stored for several years at room temperature without significant physical change or loss of biological activity (Pingel and Vølund, 1972).

The progressive propensity of insulin in solution to aggregate and form precipitates, however, has been noted by many investigators working with continuous insulin infusion from delivery devices (Lougheed et al., 1980; Buchwald et al., 1980), especially when the pump design is based upon a peristaltic system (Irsigler and Kritz, 1979, Jackman et al., 1980; Prestele, Franetzki, and Kresse, 1980; James et al., 1981). This precipitation problem is a major impediment to safe clinical application of implantable insulin delivery systems.

The inherent tendency of insulin to form aggregates or fibrils by non-covalent polymerization (Waugh et al., 1953) is promoted by a combination of physical factors, such as heat, movement, and hydrophobic surfaces; therefore, present commercial insulin solutions are not sufficiently stable for long-term use in implantable infusion systems.

This article presents data on how purity of insulin and composition of insulin solution influence physical and chemical stability of insulin. Furthermore, requirements for introducing fibrillation-inhibiting additives and possibilities of improving physical stability by these means are described. Finally, preliminary results are presented with respect to the influence of different materials used for pump construction on physical stability of insulin solutions.

Materials and Methods

Commercial insulin solutions of different brands were obtained from the wholesaler or drug store and examined two to seven months after manufacture according to the expiration date. The b-component (Steiner *et al.*, 1968) was prepared by pooling and lyophilization of fractions, obtained after gel filtration on Sephadex G 50 of first crystals of porcine insulin.

Porcine proinsulin was prepared as described by Heding *et al.* (1974). The non-convertible dimer was prepared from porcine b-component by anion-exchange chromatography slightly modified after Jørgensen *et al.* (1970). An ion strength of 0.13 and a pH of 8.4 were used for the eluent.

All other chemicals used were of pharmacopoeial or analytical grade.

Analysis by gel filtration (content of covalent polymerization products and of a- and b-components) was performed as described by Schlichtkrull *et al.* (1974).

Physical stability was evaluated by shaking normal insulin vials (diameter 1.8 cm, height 6.5 cm) at an elevated temperature. Five vials containing the test sample (10 ml) were placed vertically in a shaking bath (Heto, Birkeroed, Denmark) and subjected to horizontal rocking movements with a frequency and amplitude of 100 min^{-1} and 50 mm, respectively. Opalescence of the test samples was monitored on a nephelometer (Fischer, type DRT 100, Bolton, Canada) with an adapter for vials. Time of fibrillation is defined as the time elapsed until the samples develop a turbidity of 10 units (NTU).

Physical compatibility with materials was evaluated as follows: A sheet of the material was cut into small, regular pieces (0.5 $\times$ 1.5 cm). After sonification, 18 cm^2 was placed in each normal insulin vial. Before closing, the vial was evacuated stepwise (0.3 and 0.1 atm for 20 min) and filled entirely with insulin solution. Several vials were subjected to alternating rotation around principal axis at 37° C (2.0 rounds/period, 43 periods/min), and turbidity was measured as described above.

Immunization experiments were carried out as described by Schlichtkrull *et al.* (1974).

Insulin absorption studies were carried out as described by Sestoft *et al.* (1982).

Results and Discussion

Chemical stability with regard to the formation of covalent di- and polymerization products of insulin is illustrated in Figure 1. Various batches of two different insulin formulations were examined by gel filtration after storage for one year at 25° C. In the formulation with NaCl and methylparaben (the original British Pharmacopoeia formulation), the mean transformation amounted to 0.8%. In the USP formulation, insulin transformation varied more from batch to batch, especially between different brands of insulin; the mean transformation was approximately four times higher than in the BP formulation.

Physical stability of insulin solutions can be evaluated in several ways. As our standard method, we have used shaking of insulin vials placed in vertical position at elevated temperature.

Table 1 compares the two pharmacopeial formulations. That the physical stability of the USP formulation appears to be substantially better than that of the BP formulation probably is due to the higher ion strength of the latter.

Physical stability also has been found to decrease with increasing purity of insulin. This is probably not a result of a deleterious effect of the purification process as such, but of the impurities present, as illustrated in Figure 2.

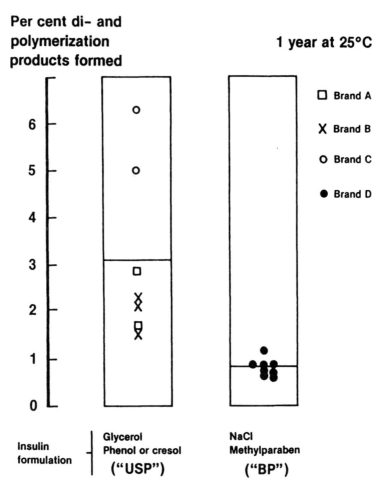

Per cent di- and polymerization products formed

1 year at 25°C

- □ Brand A
- X Brand B
- O Brand C
- ● Brand D

| Insulin formulation | Glycerol Phenol or cresol ("USP") | NaCl Methylparaben ("BP") |

Figure 1. Formation of covalent di- and polymerization products during storage of neutral insulin solutions.

Table 1. Comparison of two pharmacopeial formulations of neutral insulin solution with respect to physical stability against fibrillation of insulin; Figures shown are means of five estimates on two and four batches, respectively

Formulation	Days to start of precipitation at 37° C
BP	0.5
USP	2.7

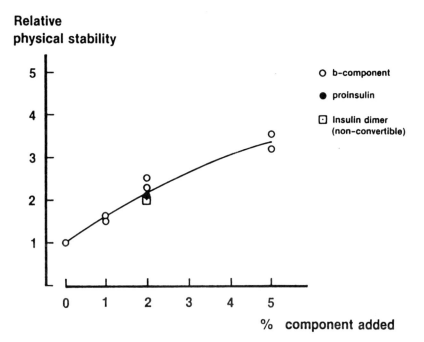

Figure 2. Physical stabilization (tested at 37° C) of neutral insulin solutions (USP formulation) by addition of different insulin-related impurities.

Some of the high molecular weight impurities, which are removed during purification, are added to monocomponent insulin. It appears that addition of the b-component enables reinstitution of physical stability. Correlation between relative physical stability, as judged by the shaking test, and the amount of impurities present is obvious.

Two main constituents of the b-component, proinsulin and the non-convertible dimer, are both as effective as the b-component mixture, and probably other insulin-like ingredients of impure insulin are likely to inhibit insulin fibrillation as well.

Differences in physical stability also have been observed between different brands of neutral solutions. Figure 3 illustrates that such variability can be explained, at least partially, by differences in purity of insulin. Three brands of highly purified insulin, each represented by two or three different batches of neutral insulin U 100 from the U. S. market, were compared with respect to physical stability and content of a- and b-component as estimated by gel filtration. Correlation between physical stability and content of high molecular weight impurities is evident.

Since more than ten years have been devoted to eliminating immunological and other untoward effects of impurities contaminating therapeutic insulin, it would be a major step backward to accept a compromise as a solution to the problem of physical stability in delivery devices.

The clinical benefits of using insulin effectively freed from impurities have been clearly demonstrated, most recently by Pietri and Raskin (1981), who

Physical stability
(days to fibrillation at 37°C)

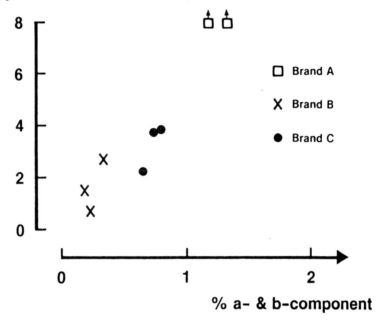

Figure 3. Physical stability versus content of a- and b-component of different brands of USP neutral insulin solutions in U 100 strength.

compared two brands of highly purified insulin and found that local allergic skin reactions occurred during continuous subcutaneous infusion in the majority of patients treated with a particular brand of insulin. The authors discuss whether differences in parts per million of impurities account for the observed difference in allergic manifestations. However, from Figure 3, it appears that differences in content of impurities also can be measured in the order of percentage.

Improvements in physical stability of neutral insulin solutions by using various fibrillation-inhibiting additives have been reported (Buchwald *et al.*, 1981; Irsigler *et al.*, 1981, Brange and Havelund, 1982b). The introduction of additives requires that the substance be physiologically acceptable and compatible not only with the insulin and auxilliary substances, but with materials used for construction of pump fluid systems. Furthermore, materials must not negatively influence insulin quality (chemical stability, timing, and immunogenicity).

Unfortunately, most additives reported to improve physical stability have been found to impair chemical and biological stability of insulin. This applies to different carbohydrates (Brange and Havelund, 1982b), as well as to glycerol, which is currently used in clinical practice with implanted pump systems (Buchwald *et al.*, 1981).

Table 2. Formation of covalent di- and polymerization products during 1 month of storage at 37° C of neutral insulin solutions (USP formulation) physically stabilized by addition of glycerol

Additive	Conc. (%)	Percent di- and polymerization products formed (1 month at 37° C)
	75	16.1%
Glycerol	90	18.1%
	96	23.9%

Table 2 shows our results from an examination by gel filtration of the effect of addition of high concentrations of glycerol on chemical stability with regard to formation of covalent polymerization products of insulin. With all glycerol concentrations tested, insulin appears to polymerize to an unacceptable degree.

We have recently (Brange and Havelund, 1982a) reported the successful use of low concentrations of Ca ions for improving physical stability without affecting quality of insulin. Figure 4 summarizes our results with different insulin concentrations. Relative physical stability, as measured in our standard test at 41° C, increases with insulin concentration and with increasing amounts of Ca ions. If Ca^{++} concentration is increased above a certain level, dependent on insulin concentration, precipitation of Ca-insulin complexes will occur during normal storage.

Our observation that Ca ions can stabilize insulin solutions is probably explained by specific binding of Ca within the zinc-insulin hexamer, which we suggest is able to protect and stabilize the hexameric structure. Such a binding site has been identified by Sudmeier *et al.* (1981). Figure 5 shows that stabilization of the hexamer by Ca^{++} does not influence rate of absorption after subcutaneous injection. As shown in Figure 6, Ca-stabilized insulin solutions have also been tested in rabbit immunization experiments and found not to be significantly immunogenic.

The incompatibility of insulin with materials used for pump construction represents another major obstacle to safe application of implanted infusion devices. Table 3 shows results of preliminary tests of the influence of different materials on the tendency of insulin to fibrillate. Silicone rubber and polypropylene with the same surface area are compared in a physical stress test in which insulin vials are exposed to alternating rotation. The two materials clearly affect the physical stability to a different degree.

Conclusion

In developing insulin preparations suitable for pump infusion, not only physical, but chemical, biological, and immunological properties, as well as material compatibility, must be considered. Addition of Ca^{++} in low concentrations offers a physiologically acceptable method of increasing physical stability of neutral insulin solutions without affecting the quality of insulin, including the timing and immunological characteristics.

Acknowledgement
The authors thank Leif Sestoft, M.D., chief physician, Hvidore Hospital, for supervising the insulin absorption studies.

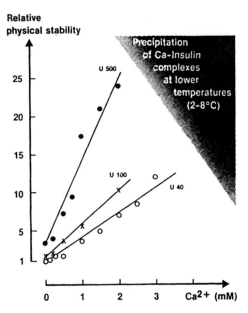

Figure 4. Effect of calcium chloride on physical stability (41° C) of neutral insulin solutions (USP formulation) of different strengths.

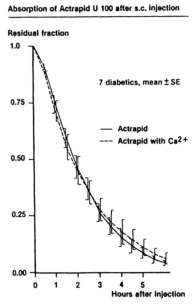

Absorption of Actrapid U 100 after s.c. injection

Figure 5. Absorption from thigh after s.c. injection of 8 i.u. of Actrapid with and without addition of 2 mM calcium chloride.

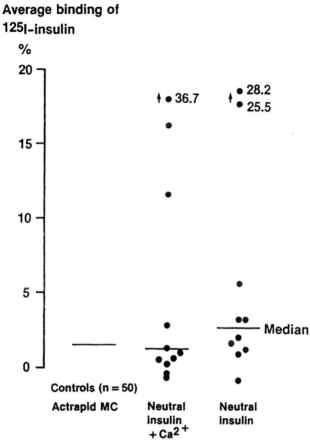

Figure 6. Groups of rabbits immunized twice weekly for three months, 20 units per injection, with Freund's incomplete adjuvant. Percent binding (area under curve) for each rabbit divided by number of days of immunization. Final serum dilution 1:3.

Table 3. Compatibility of neutral insulin solution (USP) with surface of various materials

Material	Days to start of insulin fibrillation (rotation at 37° C)
Glass	> 200
Glass + Silicone rubber	3-5
Glass + Polypropylene	17-21

References

Brange J, Havelund S (1982a). Properties of insulin in solution. *In* Proceedings from the International Symposium on Artificial Systems for Insulin Delivery. Assisi, Sept. 1981. Raven Press (in press).

Brange J, Havelund S (1982b). Insulin pumps and insulin quality—requirements and problems. *Acta Med Scand.* (in press).

Buchwald H, Rohde TD, Dorman FD, Skakoon JG, Wigness BD, Prosl FR, Tucker EM, Rublein TG, Blackshear PJ, Varco RL (1980). A totally implantable drug infusion device: laboratory and clinical experience using a model with single flow rate and new design for modulated insulin infusion. *Diabetes Care* 3:351-8.

Buchwald H, Varco RL, Rupp WM, Goldenberg FJ, Barbosa J, Rohde TD, Schwartz RA, Rublein TG, Blackshear PJ (1981). Treatment of a type II diabetic by a totally implantable insulin infusion device. *Lancet* 2:1233-4.

Heding LG, Larsen UD, Markussen J, Jørgensen KH, Hallund O (1974). Radioimmunoassays for human, pork and ox C-peptides and related substances. *Horm Metab Res Suppl Ser.* 5:40-4.

Irsigler K, Kritz H (1979). Long-term continuous intravenous insulin therapy with a portable insulin dosage-regulating apparatus. *Diabetes* 28:196-203.

Irsigler K, Kritz H, Hagmüller G, Franetzki M, Prestele K, Thurow H, Geisen K (1981). Long-term continuous intraperitoneal insulin infusion with an implanted remote-controlled insulin infusion device. *Diabetes* 30:1072-5.

Jackman WS, Lougheed W, Marliss EB, Zinman B, Albisser AM (1980). For insulin infusion: a miniature precision peristaltic pump and silicone rubber reservoir. *Diabetes Care* 3:322-31.

James DE, Jenkins AB, Kraegen EW, Chisholm DJ (1981). Insulin precipitation in artificial infusion devices. *Diabetologia* 21:554-7.

Jørgensen, KH, Brange J, Hallund O, Pingel M (1970). A method for the preparation of essentially pure insulin. *In* International Congress Series No. 209. VII Congress of the International Diabetes Federation (RR Rodrigues, FJG Ebling, I Henderson, R Assan, eds.). Amsterdam, Excerpta Medica Foundation. Abstracts, p. 149.

Lougheed WD, Woulfe-Flanagan H, Clement JR, Albisser AM (1980). Insulin aggregation in artificial delivery systems. *Diabetologia* 19:1-19.

Pietri A, Raskin P (1981). Cutaneous complications of chronic continuous subcutaneous infusion therapy. *Diabetes Care* 4:624-6.

Pingel M, Vølund Aa (1972). Stability of insulin preparations. *Diabetes* 21:805-13.

Prestele K, Franetzki M, Kresse H (1980). Development of program-controlled portable insulin delivery devices. *Diabetes Care* 3:362-8.

Schlichtkrull J, Munck O, Jersild M (1965). Insulin Rapitard and Insulin Actrapid. *Acta Med Scand.* 177:103-13.

Schlichtkrull J, Brange J, Christiansen AaH, Hallund O, Heding LG, Jørgensen KH, Rasmussen SM, Sørensen E, Vølund Aa (1974). Monocomponent insulin and its clinical implications. *Horm Metab Res Suppl Ser.* 5:134-43.

Sestoft L, Vølund Aa, Gammeltoft S, Birch K, Hildebrandt P (1982). The biological properties of human insulin. *Acta Med Scand.* (in press).

Steiner DF, Hallund O, Rubenstein A, Cho S, Bayliss C (1968). Isolation and properties of proinsulin, intermediate forms, and other minor components from crystalline bovine insulin. *Diabetes* 17:725-36.

Sudmeier JL, Bell SJ, Storm MC, Dunn MF (1981). Cadmium-113 nuclear magnetic resonance studies of bovine insulin: two-zinc insulin hexamer specifically binds calcium. *Science* 212:560-2.

Waugh DF, Wilhelmson DF, Commerford SL, Sackler ML (1953). Studies of the nucleation and growth reaction of selected types of insulin fibrils. *J Am Chem Soc.* 75:2592-2600.

Reproduced from *Diabetic Medicine*, 3:532–536, 1986. Copyright
John Wiley & Sons Ltd. 1986. With permission.

Neutral Insulin Solutions Physically Stabilized by Addition of Zn^{2+}

J. Brange[a], S. Havelund[a], E. Hommel[b], E. Sørensen[a], C. Kühl[b]

[a]*Novo Research Institute and* [b]*Hvidøre Hospital, Copenhagen, Denmark*

Commercial neutral insulin solutions, all of which contain 2–3 zinc atoms per hexameric unit of insulin, have a relatively limited physical stability when exposed to heat and movement, as for example in insulin infusion pumps. Physical stabilization of neutral insulin solutions has been obtained by addition of two extra Zn^{2+} per hexamer of insulin. This addition stabilizes porcine and human neutral solutions equally well and does not affect the chemical stability of the insulin. The stabilization is probably obtained by a further strengthening of the hexameric structure of insulin, so that the formation of insoluble insulin fibrils (via the dissociation into the insulin monomer or dimer) is impeded or prevented. The addition of an extra 2 Zn^{2+} has been shown to be without influence on the insulin immunogenicity in rabbits or on the rate of absorption after subcutaneous injection in diabetic patients. It is concluded that neutral insulin solution can be physically stabilized by addition of extra Zn^{2+} without affecting other qualities of the insulin preparation including chemical stability, immunogenicity, and duration of action after injection.

KEY WORDS Insulin Physical stability Neutral insulin solution
Subcutaneous absorption Chemical stability Immunogenicity Zinc stabilization
Insulin precipitation Insulin fibrillation

Introduction

The stability of insulin in solution has been greatly improved since its introduction in 1923. In the early years of insulin manufacture a low pH was required to solubilize the very impure insulin and to protect the insulin from degradation by contaminating pancreatic enzymes. This enzymatic degradation was further counteracted by adding Zn ions to the acid solution.[1] Later on it became possible to remove the enzymes and the overall purity of insulin was improved sufficiently to allow the manufacture of the first solution of insulin with a physiological pH.[2,3]

Commercial neutral insulin solutions contain Zn ions corresponding to 2–3 zinc atoms per hexameric unit of insulin, resulting in a predominant population of hexameric insulin molecules. This association state of the insulin represents a relatively stable unit allowing storage of pharmaceutical solutions for several years at room temperature without further aggregation and precipitation of the insulin.

These neutral solutions, however, are not sufficiently stable for long-term use in infusion pumps[4,5] because the insulin solution in such systems is exposed to a combination of relatively high temperature (30–37°C), hydrophobic surfaces, and motion. Addition of Ca^{2+} [6] or increase of the Zn ion content to 4–5 atoms Zn per hexamer[7,8] has been shown to improve the physical stability of a neutral insulin solution considerably. Thus Zn ions could again play an important role in stabilizing insulin solutions. We have studied the properties of such zinc stabilized neutral insulin solutions in terms of physical and chemical stability, immunogenicity in rabbits, and the SC absorption rate in diabetic patients.

Materials and Methods

Insulin preparations

The experimental neutral porcine or human insulin solutions were prepared from commercial Actrapid^R insulin (100 U/ml, 0.2% phenol, 1.6% glycerol, 2.3 Zn atoms per hexamer of insulin, Novo Industri) by addition of zinc acetate to obtain the specified number of Zn atoms per hexamer ($\pm$0.1), or from zinc-free sodium insulin crystals (Novo Research Institute, Copenhagen, Denmark) by addition of the same auxiliary substances.

Insulin was labelled with ^{125}I using the iodate method,[9] without subsequent chromatographic purification. The following modifications were introduced: formation of di-iodo-insulin was suppressed by using 3 mCi ^{125}I-insulin for iodination of 3 mg of insulin; a solution of 2 g/l of insulin in 0.01 mol/l HCl was used (instead of human albumin) for dissolving the precipitate to 40 mCi ^{125}I per litre; the pH of the final ^{125}I-insulin solution was adjusted to 3.5–4.5 with 1 mol/l Na acetate.

The radioactively labelled preparations for the clinical absorption studies were made by addition of an acid solution of ^{125}I-insulin to an acid solution of unlabelled homologous insulin, followed by neutralization to pH 7.4 and addition of the auxiliary substances (0.2% phenol,

Correspondence to: Dr J. Brange, Novo Research Institute, Novo Alle,
DK 2880 BAGSVAERD, Denmark.

Accepted 23 May 1986

1.6% glycerol). The composition of the four different preparations varied with respect to insulin species and Zn content. The final activity was 2–3 μCi/ml. All chemicals used were analytical grade.

Shaking Test

The physical stability of the insulin solutions was evaluated comparatively by shaking normal insulin vials (diameter 18 mm, height 65 mm) at 37°C or 41°C (±0.1°C). Vials containing the insulin solution (10 ml) and atmospheric air (3 ml) were placed vertically in a shaking bath (Heto, Birkerød, Denmark) and subjected to horizontal rocking movements with a frequency and amplitude of 100/min and 50 mm, respectively. Opalescence of the test samples was monitored on a nephelometer (Fischer, type DRT 100, Bolton, Canada) with an adapter for vials. The initial turbidity of an insulin solution is 0.3–1.5 nephelometric turbidity units (NTU)[10] dependent on the insulin concentration and the auxiliary substances used. Time of fibrillation was defined as the time elapsed until the samples develop a turbidity of 10 NTU, which corresponds to a turbidity just visible to the naked eye. The amount of insulin precipitated from a 100 U/ml preparation with NTU=10 was about 1.5% of the total insulin.

Chemical Analyses

Chemical stability of the insulin in the different formulations was evaluated by a two-step high performance liquid chromatography (HPLC) method. The first step was size exclusion chromatography (estimation of covalent di- and polymerization products of insulin) on a Waters I-125 column (8 × 300 mm); the eluent was acetic acid 2.5 mol/l, L-arginine 0.004 mol/l, acetonitrile 4%; flow rate was 0.7 ml/min; ambient temperature. In the second step the peak from the first chromatogram containing the 5000–7000 MW fraction (insulin + derivatives) was automatically transferred to a reverse phase separation on a Nucleosil C_{18} column (40 × 200 mm). Reservoir A: ammonium sulfate 0.1 mol/l, pH 2.3. Reservoir B: acetonitrile. Elution: isocratically 11 min with 26.6% B and gradient (60 min) to 32.0% B, flow 0.8 ml/min, 15°C. In the first step the eluted compounds were monitored by their absorbance at 280 nm and in the second step at 214 nm.

Immunogenicity in Rabbits

Immunization experiments were carried out in rabbits as described by Schlichtkrull et al.[11] with the exception that complete Freund's adjuvant was used in the first injection.

Timing

The absorption study comprised six insulin-treated diabetic patients (two females and four males) aged 22 to 44 years (mean 31 years). Their daily insulin dose ranged from 36 to 48 U (mean 43 U). Three patients had background retinopathy, one had mild nephropathy and one incipient peripheral neuropathy. None had lipodystrophy at injection sites. Informed consent was obtained from each patient before the study, which was approved by the local ethical committee.

The method used to study insulin absorption was local external counting of the residual raidoactivity of injected ^{125}I-labelled insulin Actrapid (with or without addition of extra Zn^{2+}). The radioactivity at the injection sites was measured by external 2 × 2 inch NaI scintillation detectors, with lead pinhole collimators fixed 60 mm above the skin surface.

The patients reported to the hospital on two different days, each day after overnight fasting. Thyroid function was blocked by administration of 200 mg potassium iodide in the morning prior to starting the investigation. Each day the absorption of two different insulin preparations was evaluated in each patient. The insulin solutions were injected subcutaneously at an angle of 45° into each thigh according to a balanced randomized plan, 8 units of one insulin being injected into one thigh and 8 units of another solution into the other thigh. Altogether four different insulin preparations were compared in each patient. The background activity was counted before each injection.

The counting was continuous except at mealtimes. Counting was terminated when residual activity was less than 10% of the initial activity (after approximately 7 h). Time until the original counts had decreased to 50% (T_{50}) was determined from the individual disapperance curves.

Statistical Methods

The differences in clinical absorption of 2 Zn and 4 Zn insulin (T_{50} values) were evaluated by analysis of variance using a 5% significance level. In the immunogenicity studies the binding of ^{125}I-insulin was compared by means of the two sample rank sum test (Mann-Whitney test).

Results

The influence of increasing amounts of Zn^{2+} on the physical stability of neutral porcine insulin solution is illustrated in Figure 1. A slight improvement in stability was seen when the Zn^{2+} content was increased from 0 to 1 and from 2 to 3 Zn atoms per hexamer, whereas a much greater one was observed when the Zn^{2+} content was further raised to 4 Zn per hexamer. Addition of Zn^{2+} was equally effective with porcine and with human insulin (Figure 2).

The chemical stability of neutral insulin solutions containing 2 and 4 Zn per hexamer of insulin is compared in Table 1. There was a tendency to less di- and polymerization at 4°C with 4 Zn compared with 2 Zn per hexamer (not statistically significant), but at 37°C this

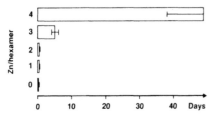

Figure 1. Physical stability of neutral porcine insulin solutions with different Zn²⁺ content in the shaking test at 37°C. Time elapsed until first visible sign of precipitation of insulin (NTU = 10, see text), mean ± SE of 4–8 samples

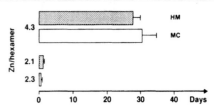

Figure 2. Physical stability of human (HM) versus porcine (MC) monocomponent Actrapid 100 U/ml with different Zn contents in the shaking test at 41°C. Time elapsed until first visible sign of precipitation of insulin (NTU = 10, see text), mean ± SE of 4 samples

Table 1. Chemical stability of insulin during storage of neutral insulin solutions with different content of Zn^{2+}, as determined by HPLC (% formed per month)

	Zn/hexamer	Species of insulin	Storage temperature 4°C	37°C
Formation of di- and polymerization products of insulin	2	human	0.027 ± 0.008	0.32 ± 0.10
		porcine	0.028 ± 0.016	0.25 ± 0.06
	4	human	0.016 ± 0.008	0.50 ± 0.17
		porcine	0.017 ± 0.007	0.32 ± 0.14
Formation of other insulin derivatives	2	human	0.11 ± 0.02	5.9 ± 0.3
		porcine	0.13 ± 0.04	6.1 ± 0.6
	4	human	0.14 ± 0.03	4.5 ± 1.1
		porcine	0.15 ± 0.06	5.3 ± 0.8

Mean ± SD of 4–6 different batches of each type.
No differences between species or zinc content were statistically significant.

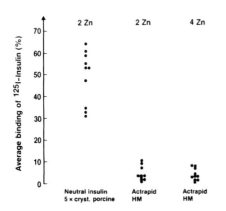

Figure 3. Groups of 10 rabbits were immunized for 100 days with 20 U insulin twice a week. First injection with Freund's complete adjuvant, following injections twice a week with incomplete adjuvant. Blood samples were drawn every 2 weeks. Per cent average binding (area under the curve) to added ¹²⁵I-insulin is calculated for each rabbit and divided by number of days of immunization. Final serum dilution 1:3. The statistical analysis showed no significant difference in antibody formation between 2 and 4 Zn Actrapid, whereas the more impure 5 times crystallized insulin is significantly ($p<0.001$) more immunogenic

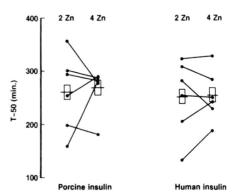

Figure 4. Absorption from the thigh after subcutaneous injection of 8 U of different 100 U/ml ¹²⁵I-labelled neutral insulin solutions in 6 diabetic patients. The standard error was obtained from the analysis of variance and represents the within-patient standard error of the means. Statistical analysis showed no significant differences in T_{50} values between 2 and 4 Zn preparations

difference was not seen. The formation of other derivatives comprising mainly products deamidated in residue B3[12] was not different in the two types of preparation.

The outcome of the rabbit immunization experiment is shown in Figure 3, which shows that antibody formation in rabbits injected with zinc stabilized neutral insulin was very low and not significantly different from that seen after injection of a neutral insulin solution with normal Zn content, whereas significantly higher ($p<0.001$) antibody titres were observed in the rabbits injected with insulin of conventional purity.

The result of the absorption study is illustrated in Figure 4. Statistical analysis showed no significant heterogeneity between patients in absorption of 2 Zn relative to 4 Zn preparations. Furthermore, there were no significant mean differences between 2 and 4 Zn preparations, neither within each insulin species nor for both species combined.

Discussion

Physical Stability

Conventional neutral insulin solutions are physically rather unstable, irrespective of insulin species and brand, when they are exposed to shaking at near-physiological temperatures. Solutions containing the most impure insulin are the most stable preparations.[13]

Many different ways of increasing the physical stability of insulin for use in infusion pumps have been reported. These methods include the use of organic medium,[14] introduction of organic[15–21] or inorganic additives,[13] and the use of insulin derivatives.[22]

Only a few of these methods are effective without compromising the quality of the insulin preparation; glycerol or carbohydrates, for example, have been found to impair the chemical and biological stability of the insulin.[13,19] The addition of surface active substances[18,21] acts by preventing the adsorption of insulin to certain hydrophobic interphases,[18] in particular the interphase to air, and therefore such additives are effective especially when the insulin solution is in contact with a certain volume of air.

Thurow and Geisen[18] have stated the effect of zinc ions to be inadequate, but this claim is based on a zinc content of 28 μg per 400 IU corresponding to 1 Zn atom per hexamer of insulin,[17] which, as seen in Figure 1, only slightly improves the stability compared with zinc-free solutions. A zinc content of 4–5 Zn^{2+} per hexamer is necessary in order to obtain a pronounced stabilizing effect.

Based on sedimentation equilibrium experiments Jeffrey[23] found the average molecular weight of insulin in neutral solution to increase slightly when the zinc content was raised from 2 to 3–4 atoms of zinc per hexamer. In addition to the two central zinc ions coordinated to histidyl B_{10} side chains[24] relatively strong binding of Zn^{2+} can occur between two B_{13} glutamic acid side chains paired together by the association of insulin dimers in the hexamer.[25] In total, three extra Zn^{2+} can be bound to the six B_{13} residues, which are at the hexamer centre, neutralizing the negative charges and most likely leading to a more stable hexameric structure. This stabilization combined with the shift to a species of relatively higher molecular weight may explain why formation of insulin fibrils, which proceeds via monomers or dimers,[26–28] is impeded when extra Zn^{2+} is added.

As in the case of conventional neutral solutions[6] and Ca^{2+}-stabilized preparations,[13] the physical stability of zinc stabilized preparations increases with increasing insulin concentration. The relative physical stability of insulin solutions containing 4 Zn per hexamer of insulin increases by a factor of 7 as estimated in the shaking test when the strength is increased from 40 U/ml to 500 U/ml.[8]

The stabilizing effect of Zn^{2+} can be obtained with other combinations of auxiliary substances. Thus phenol can be substituted by, for example, m-cresol or methylparaben and glycerol by NaCl.

In an experimental implantable insulin pump (IPIP)[29] tested during simulated in vivo conditions (37°C, gentle shaking) a zinc stabilized 500 U/ml preparation has proven physically stable for more than 2 years of continuous pumping.

Absorption rate and Immunogenicity

As insulin is assumed to be absorbed from the subcutaneous tissue in a dimeric or monomeric state[30] one would expect that stabilization of the hexameric unit would lead to a slower disappearance from the injection site. This was not the case in the present study, probably because the dissociation of the hexamer is not the rate limiting step in the absorption process. The trial design with 12 injections each of a 2 Zn and a 4 Zn preparation does not exclude that a minor difference in absorption rate exists (type 2 error). However, the 95% confidence interval for the difference in T_{50}, based on the t-distribution, is ±16%, and this difference is small compared with normal day-to-day variations.

The low immunogenicity in rabbits of 2 Zn neutral MC or HM Actrapid is not influenced by the additional Zn ions. Similar results with respect to absorption rate and immunogenicity were obtained with Ca^{2+}-stabilized porcine neutral insulin solutions.[13]

Acknowledgements

The authors wish to thank Dr Aa. Vølund for statistical evaluation of the data and L. Grønlund Andersen for excellent technical assistance.

References

1. Sahyun M, Nixon A, Goodell M. Influence of certain metals on the stability of insulin. *J Pharmacol Exp Ther* 1939; **65:** 143–149.
2. Schlichtkrull J, Funder J, Munck O. Clinical evaluation of a new insulin preparation. In: *4e Congrès de la Fédération Internationale du Diabète, Genève,* Demole M (Ed.). Genève: Éditions Mèdecine et Hygiène, 1961; **I:** 303–305.
3. Schlichtkrull J, Munck O, Jersild M. Insulin Rapitard and Insulin Actrapid. *Acta Med Scand* 1965; **177:** 103–113.
4. Lougheed WD, Woulfe-Flanagan H, Clement JR, Albisser AM. Insulin aggregation in artificial delivery systems. *Diabetologia* 1980; **19:** 1–9.
5. James DE, Jenkins AB, Kraegen EW, Chisholm DJ. Insulin precipitation in artificial infusion devices. *Diabetologia* 1981; **21:** 554–557.
6. Brange J, Havelund S. Properties of insulin in solution. In: *Artificial Systems for Insulin Delivery,* Brunetti P, Alberti KGMM, Albisser AM, Hepp KD, Benedetti MM (Eds). New York: Raven Press, 1983, 83–88.
7. Brange J, Havelund S. United States patent no 4,476,118, 1984.
8. Brange J, Skelbæk-Pedersen B, Langkjær L et al. Galenics of insulin preparations. In: *Subcutaneous Insulin Therapy,* Berger M (Ed.) Springer-Verlag Heidelberg.
9. Jørgensen KH, Larsen UD. Homogeneous mono-^{125}I-insulins. Preparation and characterization of mono-[125]I-(Tyr A14)-and mono-[125]I-(Tyr A19)-insulin. *Diabetologia* 1980; **19:** 546–554.
10. Rice EW. The preparation of formazin standards for nephelometry. *Anal Chim Acta* 1976; **87:** 251–253.
11. Schlichtkrull J, Brange J, Christiansen AaH et al. Monocomponent insulin and its clinical implications. *Horm Metab Res* 1974; (suppl Ser) **5:** 134–143.
12. Brange J, Langkjær L, Havelund S, Sørensen E. Chemical stability of insulin: Neutral insulin solutions. *Diabetologia* 1983; **25:**193 (abstract).
13. Brange J, Havelund S, Hansen PE, Langkjær L, Sørensen E, Hildebrandt P. Formulation of physically stable neutral insulin solutions for continuous infusion by delivery systems. In: *Hormone Drugs,* Gueriguian JL, Bransome ED, Outschoorn AS (Eds). FDA–USP Workshop, Bethesda, Md, USA, May 19–21, 1982. The United States Pharmacopeial Convention Inc., Rockville, 1982: 92–105.
14. Blackshear PJ, Rohde TD, Palmer JL et al. Glycerol prevents insulin precipitation and interruption of flow in an implantable insulin infusion pump. *Diabetes Care* 1983; **6:** 387–392.
15. Quinn R, Andrade JD. Minimizing the aggregation of neutral insulin solutions. *J Pharm Sci* 1983; **72:** 1472–1473.
16. Sato S, Ebert CD, Kim SW. Prevention of insulin self-association and surface adsorption. *J Pharm Sci* 1983; **72:** 228–232.
17. Thurow H. Studies on the denaturation of dissolved insulin. In: *Insulin, chemistry, structure and function of insulin and related hormones.* Brandenburg D, Wollmer A (Eds). Berlin, New York: Walter de Gruyter, 1980, 215–221.
18. Thurow H, Geisen K. Stabilization of dissolved proteins against denaturation at hydrophobic interfaces. *Diabetologia* 1984; **27:** 212–218.
19. Brange J, Havelkund S. Insulin pumps and insulin quality – requirements and problems. *Acta Med Scand* 1983; Suppl. **671:** 135–138.
20. Bringer J, Heldt A, Grodsky GM. Prevention of insulin aggregation by dicarboxylic amino acids during prolonged infusion. *Diabetes* 1981; **30:** 83–85.
21. Chawla AS, Hinberg I, Blais P, Johnson D. Aggregation of insulin, containing surfactants, in contact with different materials. *Diabetes* 1985; **34:** 420–424.
22. Albisser AM, Williamson JR, Lougheed WD. Desired characteristics of insulins to be used in infusion pumps. In: *Hormone Drugs,* (see ref. 13 pp 84–95).
23. Jeffrey PD. Ploymerization behaviour of bovine zinc-insulin at neutral pH. Molecular weight of the subunit and the effect of glucose. *Biochemistry* 1974; **13:** 4441–4447.
24. Adams MJ, Blundell TL, Dodson EJ et al. Structure of rhombohedral 2 zinc insulin crystals. *Nature* 1969; **224:** 491–495.
25. Emdin SO, Dodson GG, Cutfield JM, Cutfield SM. Role of zinc in insulin biosynthesis. Some possible zinc-insulin interactions in the pancreatic B-cell. *Diabetologia* 1980; **19:** 174–182.
26. Waugh DF, Wilhelmson DF, Commerford SL, Sackler ML. Studies of the nucleation and growth reactions of selected types of insulin fibrils. *J Am Chem Soc* 1953; **75:** 2592–2600.
27. Koltun WL, Waugh DF, Bear RS. An X-ray diffraction investigation of selected types of insulin fibrils. *J Am Chem Soc* 1954; **76:** 413–417.
28. Burke MJ, Rougvie MA. Cross-B protein structures. I. Insulin fibrils. *Biochemsitry* 1972; **11:** 2435–2439.
29. Fischell RE, Radford WE, Saudek CD. A programmable implantable medication system: application to diabetes. In: *Proceedings of the 16th Hawaii International Conference on System Sciences,* January 6–9, 1983. USA: Western Periodicals Co, 1983, 2:229–234.
30. Binder C. A theoretical model for the absorption of soluble insulin. In: *Artificial Systems for Insulin Delivery,* Brunetti P, Alberti KGMM, Albisser AM, Hepp KD, Benedetti MM (Eds). New York: Raven Press, 1983, 53–57.

Reproduced from *Pharmaceutical Research*, 9(6):715–726, 1992.

Research Article

Chemical Stability of Insulin. 1. Hydrolytic Degradation During Storage of Pharmaceutical Preparations

Jens Brange,[1,2] Liselotte Langkjær,[1] Svend Havelund,[1] and Aage Vølund[1]

Received August 8, 1991; accepted December 22, 1991

Hydrolysis of insulin has been studied during storage of various preparations at different temperatures. Insulin deteriorates rapidly in acid solutions due to extensive deamidation at residue Asn^{A21}. In neutral formulations deamidation takes place at residue Asn^{B3} at a substantially reduced rate under formation of a mixture of isoAsp and Asp derivatives. The rate of hydrolysis at B3 is independent of the strength of the preparation, and in most cases the species of insulin, but varies with storage temperature and formulation. Total transformation at B3 is considerably reduced when insulin is in the crystalline as compared to the amorphous or soluble state, indicating that formation of the rate-limiting cyclic imide decreases when the flexibility of the tertiary structure is reduced. Neutral solutions containing phenol showed reduced deamidation probably because of a stabilizing effect of phenol on the tertiary structure (α-helix formation) around the deamidating residue, resulting in a reduced probability for formation of the intermediate imide. The ratio of isoAsp/Asp derivative was independent of time and temperature, suggesting a pathway involving only intermediate imide formation, without any direct side-chain hydrolysis. However, increasing formation of Asp relative to isoAsp derivative was observed with decreasing flexibility of the insulin three-dimensional structure in the formulation. In certain crystalline suspensions a cleavage of the peptide bond A8–A9 was observed. Formation of this split product is species dependent: bovine > porcine > human insulin. The hydrolytic cleavage of the peptide backbone takes place only in preparations containing rhombohedral crystals in addition to free zinc ions.

KEY WORDS: insulin; chemical stability; deamidation; hydrolysis; autocatalysis; chain cleavage.

INTRODUCTION

Insulin has been in therapeutic use for 70 years but its stability in pharmaceutical formulations has so far been studied systematically only in terms of biological potency (1,2). Little information has appeared in the literature on the chemical transformation of insulin during storage of insulin preparations, and most studies have dealt with the hydrolysis in acid medium into insulin desamido products (3,4). Decomposition of insulin during storage of bovine insulin in solid state has been studied by Fisher and Porter (5). Today virtually all insulin preparations are neutral solutions or suspensions in which deamidation occurs at a much slower rate (6,7).

Insulin has been formulated into many different pharmaceutical preparations varying with respect to type (timing characteristics), which differ as to exact formulation and composition (for review see Ref. 8). However, very little has been reported about the influence of formulation and composition on the chemical stability of insulin during storage of the preparations.

Until the late 1960s crystalline insulin was considered essentially pure insulin, but the introduction of new analytical methods made it possible to detect the presence of significant amounts of protein impurities by disc electrophoresis and gel filtration. The purity of recrystallized insulin as revealed by these methods was only 80–90% (8), rendering exact assessment of chemical stability extremely difficult. Therefore, a prerequisite for the present studies has been the introduction of monocomponent (MC) insulins (9) which are, by chromatographic methods, purified to the extent that impurities are virtually undetectable by the above methods.

The purpose of our studies was to investigate the degradation or transformation of insulin during storage of pharmaceutical preparations, using disc electrophoresis, size exclusion chromatography (SEC), and HPLC.

We report here on the quantitative aspects of the hydrolytic deterioration of insulin during storage of different preparations whereas the chemical transformation into higher molecular weight products is communicated in a subsequent paper (10).

Proteins are known to be degraded nonenzymatically by various chemical reactions (11). The most prevalent of these is deamidation, a reaction in which the side-chain amide group in glutaminyl or asparaginyl residues is hydrolyzed to form a free carboxylic acid (12,13). Insulin contains six such residues, Gln^{A5}, Gln^{A15}, Asn^{A18}, Asn^{A21}, Asn^{B3}, and Gln^{B4}

[1] Novo Research Institute, Novo Alle, DK-2880 Bagsvaerd, Denmark.
[2] To whom correspondence should be addressed at Novo Research Institute, Novo Alle, DK-2880 Bagsvaerd, Denmark.

(Fig. 1A), of which the three asparagine residues (Figs. 1A and B) are likely to be the most labile sites (12), in particular the C-terminal residue A21 upon acid treatment (3,4).

The preparations studied are listed in Table I together with their naming in different major pharmacopoeias and the abbreviations used in the text. The compositions of these preparations appear in Table II. Preliminary accounts have been published in abstract form (14,15) and in excerpt (8).

MATERIALS AND METHODS

Chemicals

Insulins used for the pharmaceutical preparations were monocomponent (MC) insulins of different species (porcine, bovine, and human) with the following characteristics: potency, 28 IU/mg (dry weight), corresponding to 1.68×10^8 IU/mol; Zn^{2+} content, 0.4%; and insulin, >99% by RP-HPLC. The content of impurities was as follows: (a) desamidoinsulins, nondetectable (<0.2%) by disc electrophoresis; and (b) di- and polymerization products, <0.2% as detected by size exclusion chromatography.

Distilled water was used for the preparation of electrophoretic buffers and chromatographic eluents. All other chemicals used were either official (Ph. Eur. or BP) or analytical grade. Porcine proinsulin was obtained from Ole Hallund, Novo Research Institute.

A

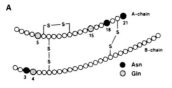

B

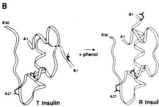

T Insulin   R Insulin

Fig. 1. Structures of insulin. (A) Primary structure of insulin shown schematically, with indications of the amino acid residues prone to deamidation. (B) Ribbon drawings of the tertiary structure (backbone) of the insulin monomer in its so-called 2 Zn structure (T Insulin) and in the phenol-induced "6 Zn" structure (R insulin) showing the most labile amide side chains (Asn residues). The view is approximately perpendicular to the crystallographic two-fold axis. It appears that the most dramatic change in the T → R structure transformation is the formation of an α-helix at the N terminal end of the B chain. This change also involves a large movement of the N terminal residues.

Manufacture

Preparation of the different formulations was performed according to the various pharmacopoeias (Table I). The types of preparations studied together with their content of auxiliary substances are listed in Table II. The majority of batches was from the production line of Novo Industri A/S, but batches produced on a smaller scale in the laboratory were also studied. Within a few days after filling into 10-ml vials samples were stored protected from light in different-temperature environments thermostatically controlled within ±1°C.

Insulin preparations from other manufacturers were purchased from drug stores and showed at least 1-year residual shelf lives.

Isolation and Storage of Samples

At appropriate intervals, 1-ml homogeneous samples were withdrawn from the vials and pH measured. Samples containing insulin in solution were adjusted to pH 6, zinc acetate (pH 6) was added to 0.01 M, and the samples were allowed to stand at 4°C overnight for complete precipitation of insulin and derivatives. Samples containing insulin solely in suspension were isolated by centrifugation, as were materials precipitated from solutions. Supernatants from suspensions as well as from precipitates were randomly controlled for derivatives appearing in solution (testing with ninhydrin). The amount was always below 0.2%. The isolated material was stored, without drying, at below −18°C until analysis.

Quantification

The studies were initiated in the early 1970s and concluded in the late 1980s, therefore the analytical techniques used have changed during the studies along with the development of modern high-performance liquid chromatographic (HPLC) methods. Initially a combination of polyacrylamide disc electrophoresis (PAGE) and densitometric scanning was used for separation and quantification. During the last 10 years HPLC has also been used.

Disc electrophoresis was performed as described earlier (9), with the following modifications: 2.5 ml of small-pore gel solution and 0.2 ml of spacer gel solution were used per column (140 × 5 mm); 10–200 μg of protein was applied (with double-constriction micropipettes) in 50 μl of spacer buffer containing 8 M urea and 0.02% (w/v) porcine proinsulin as an internal standard. The samples were run in two to four concentrations to ensure that the amounts of insulin and its derivatives were within the linear part of the standard curves (2–15 μg; see Densitometry). Electrophoresis was continued at 3 mA per column until 10 min after the tracker dye (bromphenol blue) reached the bottom of the gels. Staining was performed in 1% amido black in 7% acetic acid for 20 hr. The gels were destained, protected from light, by diffusion in 3% acetic acid for 5 days, with change of destainer three times per day. The gels with different dilutions of the same sample were destained in the same container. The stained gels were kept at room temperature in the dark until scanning, which was performed within 14 days after staining.

Table I. Types of Insulin Preparations

Classification after timing of action	Name of Preparation	Abbreviation used in text	Pharmacopoeia name		
			USP	BP	Ph. Eur.
Rapid-acting	Acid regular	Regular A	Insulin injection	Acid insulin injection	Insulini solutio iniectabilis
	Neutral regular	Regular N		Insulin injection	
Short-acting	Insulin zinc suspension, amorphous	IZS amorph.	Prompt insulin zinc suspension	Insulin zinc suspension (amorphous)	Insulini zinci amorphi suspensio iniectabilis
Intermediate-acting	Insulin zinc suspension, mixed	IZS mixed	Insulin zinc suspension	Insulin zinc suspension	Insulini zinci suspensio iniectabilis mixta
	Isophane insulin (NPH)[a]	NPH	Isophane insulin suspension	Isophane insulin injection	Insulini isophani protaminati suspensio iniectabilis
Long-acting	Insulin zinc suspension, crystalline	IZS cryst.	Extended insulin zinc suspension	Insulin zinc suspension (crystalline)	Insulini zinci cristallisati suspensio iniectabilis
	Protamine zinc insulin	PZI	Protamine zinc insulin suspension		Insulini zinci protaminati suspensio iniectabilis
Biphasic-acting	Biphasic insulin	Biphasic		Biphasic insulin injection	

[a] Neutral protamine Hagedorn.

To ensure sufficient separation of the protein bands for scanning purposes, not more than 200 μg of sample could be loaded on the disc gel. The smallest amount which could be clearly distinguished from baseline readings (see densitometry) was about 2 μg of protein, meaning that the detection limit with respect to quantitative estimation was about 1%. On the other hand, by loading larger amounts visual comparison of the test gel and standard gels allowed for a semiquantitative detection limit of about 0.2%.

Densitometry. The absorbance of the stained bands was measured on a Joyce-Loebl chromoscan (Mk II double-beam) recording densitometer (Team Valley, England) with automatic electronic integration of densitometric readings and with high-resolution transmission attachment to magnify the image of the sample. The balancing wedge ranged from 0 to 2 optical density units, the nominal wavelength of the filter at maximum transmission was 595 nm; the scanning slit was set to approx. 3×0.2 mm, and the scan expansion on the original record relative to the gel was $9\times$. The gels were placed submerged in 3% acetic acid in a quartz cuvette with a fixed distance between slit and gel. Integrator counts were corrected for baseline counts recorded cathodically to the insulin band.

The absorbance of the stained bands on the disc gels was shown to be linear at least up to 15 μg of applied insulin and of the individual desamido insulins including isoAsp B3.

On a weight basis, insulin and the desamido insulins gave identical standard curves. The densitometric readings were shown to decrease by approx. 30% during storage of the stained gel for 4 weeks. Therefore scanning of gels with different dilutions of the same sample was performed the same day and always within 1–2 weeks after destaining. Reproducibility of the results obtained after scanning of the same set of gels (same sample, different dilutions) at 1-week intervals was about ±10% (coefficient of variation, 0.11; $n = 14$), with more than 5% of derivative formed (corresponding to 10–20 μg in the band). With <10 μg in the band the variation was doubled (CV = 0.22, $n = 19$).

The relative content of the individual derivatives was calculated as the ratio of the densitometric reading of the derivative band (sample gel) to that of the insulin band (diluted sample gel, corrected for dilution factor) plus the derivative bands with adjustment for difference in internal standard readings.

HPLC. A two-step HPLC method in which the 6000 MW fraction from a separation on a size exclusion chromatography (HP-SEC) column in the second step is analyzed on a reverse-phase HPLC (RP-HPLC), as described earlier (16), was used to relate the peaks in the chromatogram to the bands on the disc gel. It appeared that the insulin di- and polymerization products removed in the first chromatographic step did not elute in the second RP-HPLC step at the

Table II. Composition of Insulin Preparations

Type of preparation[a]	Physical state of insulin[b]	pH	Auxiliary substance(s)		
			Preservative	Isotonic agent	Other additives
Regular A1	D	3	Phenol, 0.2%	Glycerol, 1.6%	
Regular A2	D	3–4	Methylparaben, 0.1%	Glucose, 5%	
Regular N1	D	7.4	Methylparaben, 0.1%	NaCl, 0.7%	Na-acetate
Regular N2	D	7.4	Phenol, 0.2%, or m-cresol 0.3%	Glycerol, 1.6%	None or Na-phosphate
Insulin zinc suspension, amorphous (IZS amorph.)	A	7.4	Methylparaben, 0.1%	NaCl, 0.7%	Zn^{2+}, Na-acetate
Insulin zinc suspension, mixed (IZS mix.)	3 parts A 7 parts C	7.4	Methylparaben, 0.1%	NaCl, 0.7%	Zn^{2+}, Na-acetate
Insulin zinc suspension, crystalline (IZS, Cryst.)	C	7.4	Methylparaben, 0.1%	NaCl, 0.7%	Zn^{2+}, Na-acetate
Isophane insulin (NPH)[c]	C	7.3	Phenol and m-cresol, total 0.3%	Glycerol, 1.6%	Protamine sulfate, Na-phosphate
Protamine zinc insulin (PZI)	A	7.3	Methylparaben, 0.1%	Glycerol, 1.6%	Protamine sulfate, Na-acetate
Biphasic insulin	1 part D (P) 3 parts C (B)	7.1	Methylparaben, 0.1%	NaCl, 0.7%	Na-acetate

[a] The abbreviations used in the text are shown in parentheses.
[b] A, amorphous; B, bovine; C, crystalline; D, dissolved; P, porcine.
[c] NPH, neutral protamine Hagedorn.

same positions as the products formed by hydrolysis, and therefore the first step has been omitted in later analyses. The RP-HPLC step was performed on a Nucleosil C_{18} column (4 × 200 mm). Reservoir A contained ammonium sulfate, 0.1 M, pH 2.3; reservoir B, acetonitrile. Elution was isocratical at 11 min, with 26% B and gradient (60 min) to 32% B; flow rate, 0.8 ml/min; and monitoring, by absorbance at 214 nm. Figure 2 illustrates the relation between the bands on the disc gel and the peaks in the HPLC chromatogram. It appears that one of the hydrolysis products (the Asp^{B3} product) is not separated from the insulin peak. However, as the ratio between the $isoAsp^{B3}$ and the Asp^{B3} products for every type of preparation has been shown within experimental error to have a fixed value for a given formulation, the value for the content of $isoAsp^{B3}$ can be used to calculate the total amount formed of the B3 transformation products.

Data Analysis

The experimental data were analyzed by polynomial regression analysis including a linear and a quadratic term: $D = a × t + b × t^2$ (D = total fraction of hydrolyzed insulin, t = time in months). This model was chosen since it describes the initial linearly increasing formation of hydrolysis product, which later on may proceed at a faster or slower rate as a consequence of pH changes in the preparations during storage. Thus the linear coefficient (a) will be an accurate estimate of the initial rate even if data at later times, when the rate of hydrolysis may have changed, are included in the regression analysis. In some cases the simple linear model appeared to be the most qualified to fit the experi-

mental data, and in a few cases (split product formation) neither of these models could be used.

Temperature coefficient Q_{10} was calculated on the basis of the expression: $\log Q_{10} = 10 × (\log k_2 - \log k_1)/(t_2 - t_1)$.

RESULTS

Three major degradation products are formed during storage of insulin solutions as revealed by disc electrophoresis, all appearing anodically to the insulin band on the gel (Fig. 3). The two bands appearing in neutral solutions of porcine (or human insulin) are different from the major band resulting from storage in acid. In neutral solutions of bovine insulin, only one band appears on the disc gel. During prolonged storage of acid solutions progressive hydrolysis and formation of desamido insulins with two or more deamidated side chains also occur (3).

It has been demonstrated (14,15) that the product in the first band anodic to insulin (R_f insulin, 1.12) is identical to monodesamido-(A21)-insulin (3). Bands 2 and 3 (R_f 1.20 and 1.26, respectively) are both deamidated in position B3, but while the upper band contains normal desamido-(B3)-insulin, the product in the lower band is isoAsp-(B3)-insulin. The single band formed during storage of bovine neutral solutions contains a mixture of the two B3 derivatives. The two B3 deamidation products can also be observed in most of the insulin suspensions after prolonged storage. In certain crystalline suspensions an additional third band (peak) arises (Fig. 2). This band (R_f 1.17 on the disc gel) contains a hydrolysis product in which the peptide linkage between amino acid residue A8 and residue A9 has been cleaved.

78

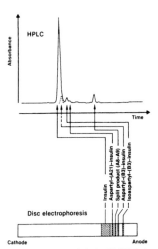

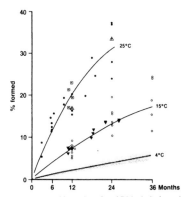

Fig. 2. Relationship between peaks in the RP-HPLC chromatogram and bands in the disc electrophoresis pattern after analysis of a pharmaceutical insulin suspension (IZS, mixed; porcine insulin) stored for 3 years at 25°C. It appears that the aspartyl-(B3)-insulin is clearly separated from insulin using disc electrophoresis, whereas the two compounds elute at approximately the same position by HPLC.

Effect of Insulin Concentration, Species, and Formulation

The rate of formation of the hydrolysis products did not vary significantly with the strength (40–400 IU/ml) for any of the preparations as exemplified in Figs. 4–6, nor could any statistical difference be observed between species of insulin (porcine, human, or bovine) with respect to formation of deamidation products (data not shown) except for preparations containing insulin zinc suspension (IZS)-type crystals. Accordingly, data on deamidation have subsequently been

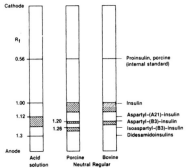

Fig. 3. Disc electrophoresis pattern of different insulin solutions (see Materials and Methods) after storage for approx. 6 months at 25°C.

Fig. 4. Time courses of formation of total B3 hydrolysis products in regular N1 insulin solutions (porcine or human insulin formulated with methylparaben + NaCl) at 4, 15, and 25°C. The curves represent the best fit of the data by polynomial regression analysis (see Materials and Methods). 4°C: Mean ± SE, $n = 20$. 15°C: Data obtained by disc electrophoresis + scanning (○); data on isoAsp[B3] formation (HPLC) transformed into total B3 transformation using the isoAsp/Asp ratios (Table III) (▼). 25°C: Data on 40 IU/ml (●); 80 IU/ml (□); 400 IU/ml (△).

pooled irrespective of the strength and, in most cases, also the species of insulin. The IZS (mixed) and the IZS crystalline formulations, however, showed significant differences between species. The rate of split product formation was

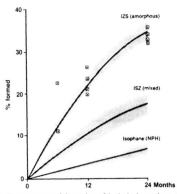

Fig. 5. Time courses of formation of hydrolysis products (mean, with 95% confidence interval hatched) during storage at 25°C of different types of pharmaceutical insulin suspensions (all formulated with porcine insulin). The curves represent the best fit of the data by polynomial regression analysis (see Materials and Methods). IZS (amorphous): 40 IU/ml ($n = 23$) + 10 results (□) on four batches with 80 or 100 IU/ml. IZS (mixed): 40 IU/ml ($n = 15$); data include split product (A8–A9) formed in the crystalline phase as well as the B3 deamidation products, which are formed mainly in the amorphous phase of the suspension. Isophane (NPH): 40 IU/ml ($n = 17$).

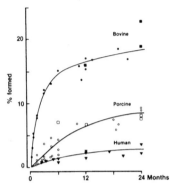

Fig. 6. Time courses of formation of the split product (A8–A9) during storage at 25°C of insulin zinc suspension, crystalline prepared from different species of insulin. Bovine: 40 IU/ml (●); 80 or 100 IU/ml (■). Porcine: 40 IU/ml (○); 80 or 100 IU/ml (□). Human: 40 IU/ml (▼).

much lower in the porcine and, especially, the human versions compared to the bovine versions of these types of preparations. To the contrary, the rate of deamidation was highest in human and negligible in bovine IZS crystalline preparations.

The composition of the acid as well as the neutral solutions had a profound influence on the rate of hydrolytic degradation of the insulin (Table III), and significant variation could also be observed between different formulations of the neutral suspensions (Table IV, Figs. 5 and 6).

Time Courses and Rate Data

Examples of the time courses of total hydrolytic degradation are given in Figs. 4 and 5. The courses with respect to formation of A8–A9 split product during storage of the long-acting crystalline Insulin Zinc Suspensions (IZS cryst.) formulated with different species of insulin are shown in Fig. 6.

The effect of temperature on such time courses of cleavage in the bovine version of this type of preparation is illustrated in Fig. 7. Large variations are observed with respect not only to the initial rate of hydrolytic degradation but also to how the degradation develops with time. The bovine IZS cryst. (Fig. 6), for example, initially degrades at a high rate, but after 12 months the rate slows down and levels off at around 20%. In contrast, the IZS amorphous (amorph.) type (Fig. 5) initially degrades at a lower rate but does not exhibit the same large reduction in the rate of formation with time.

Rate data are shown in Tables III and IV together with the ratios in which isoAsp[B3] and Asp[B3] products are formed. The rate of deamidation in neutral solution is reduced by 1 order of magnitude as compared to deamidation in acid solutions, and the rate is lower in regular N2, formulated with glycerol and phenol/cresol, than in regular N1, with NaCl and methylparaben. The initial rate of hydrolysis in neutral medium varies at 4°C from 0.3% per year in the IZS cryst. (formulated with porcine insulin) to 2.3% per year in the IZS amorph. type of formulation. At 25°C the lowest rate of formation of total hydrolysis products is seen in the NPH type (0.3% deamidation per month) and the highest rate in the IZS cryst. type formulated with bovine insulin (6% per month of mainly split product). Rate data for formation of the individual hydrolysis products in the IZS cryst. preparations are shown in Table V.

The two B3 transformation products are formed at a fixed ratio independent of temperature and time, which is in agreement with observations on succinimide formation and subsequent hydrolysis of asparaginyl residues in model peptides (13,17). The ratio is, however, influenced by composition and formulation. Thus, while the formation of the isoAsp[B3] derivative dominates in neutral solution (Table III), the Asp derivative is the main product of deamidation in the semisolid state in the neutral suspensions (Table IV).

Formation of the A8–A9 split product was observed only in the IZS types of formulations containing crystals, i.e., IZS, cryst. and mixed. Its rate of formation varies at 4°C from below the detection limit (approx. 0.05% per year) in the human insulin version to 0.6% per year in the bovine formulation. At 25°C the rates for the human, porcine, and

Table III. Formation of Insulin Deamidation Products in Pharmaceutical Insulin Solutions[a]

Insulin formulation	Temperature (°C)					Ratio isoAsp/Asp derivative
	4	15	25	37	45	
Regular A1	1.4					
	(0.1, $n = 4$)					
Regular A2	Approx. 4[b]					
Regular N1	0.18	0.65	2.10	15.3	31.0	1.9
	(0.02, $n = 20$)	(0.05, $n = 34$)	(0.16, $n = 27$)	(0.4, $n = 10$)	(0.3, $n = 11$)	
	$b = -0.07$[c]	$b = -0.43$	$b = -3.3$	$b = -250$	$b = -760$	
Regular N2	0.11	0.32	1.06	5.1	14.4	1.4
	(0.02, $n = 5$)	(0.02, $n = 7$)	(0.18, $n = 22$)	(0.2, $n = 9$)	(0.2, $n = 15$)	
			$b = -0.04$	$b = -44$	$b = -530$	

[a] The data are the apparent rate constants $k_{obs.} \times 10^2$/month (±SE).
[b] Based on data from Ref. 8.
[c] b values ($\times 10^4$)—the coefficients to the quadratic term—are given when the polynomial equation showed the best fit to the experimental data (see Materials and Methods). In all other cases the best fits are linear.

Table IV. Formation of Insulin Hydrolysis Products (Total Amounts) in Intermediate- and Long-Acting Insulin Suspensions

Type of preparation	Storage temperature (°C)[a]			Ratio isoAsp/Asp
	4	15	25	
Insulin Zinc Suspensions:				
Amorphous	0.19	0.77	2.23	0.6
	(0.02, n = 28)	(0.06, n = 15)	(0.14, n = 33)	
		$b = -1.0^b$	$b = -3.3$	
Crystalline				
Porcine	0.027	0.30	1.1[c]	0.5
	(0.006, n = 13)	(0.01, n = 10)	(0.1, n = 5)	
		$b = -0.09$		
Human	0.03	0.12	1.4[c]	0.6
	(0.01, n = 12)	(0.01, n = 8)	(0.1, n = 5)	
		$b = -0.1$		
Bovine	0.10	0.58	5.9[d]	
	(0.02, n = 14)	(0.05, n = 10)	(0.2, n = 6)	
	$b = -0.02$	$b = -0.8$		
Mixed (amorph./cryst.)				
Porcine or Human	0.10	0.32	1.0	0.6
	(0.01, n = 6)	(0.03, n = 4)	(0.2, n = 15)	
			$b = -1.2$	
Porcine/Bovine	0.12		2.0	0.6
	(0.05, n = 11)		(0.2, n = 13)	
			$b = -5$	
NPH	0.07		0.15	0.6
	(0.02, n = 7)		(0.04, n = 13)	
PZI	0.09		1.7	
	(0.02, n = 3)		(0.2, n = 5)	
			$b = -4$	
Biphasic	0.05		0.54	
	(0.02, n = 8)		(0.07, n = 17)	
			$b = -0.3$	

[a] The figures are the apparent rate constants $k_{obs.} \times 10^2$/month (±SE).
[a] The b-values ($\times 10^4$) indicate the best fit to the expression: Fraction formed = $kT + bT^2$.
[c] Linear over 1.5–6 months.
[d] Linear over 0.3–1.5 months, for time course of formation of the main hydrolysis product (A8-A9 split product) (see Fig. 6 and Table V).

bovine formulations are 0.4, 1.0, and 5.9% per month, respectively. The split product formation seems to depend not only on the type of crystals but also on the composition of the suspension. In biphasic insulin with the same rhombo-

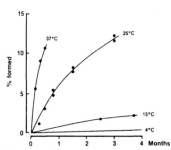

Fig. 7. Time courses of formation of the split product (A8–A9) during storage of bovine insulin zinc suspension, crystalline at different temperatures. The course at 4°C, based on results (n = 6) from 2 to 10 years of storage, corresponds to the formation of approx. 0.05% per month.

hedral crystals as in bovine IZS cryst., split product formation is virtually undetectable. These two types of preparations differ with respect to pH (7.1 versus 7.4, respectively), the content of porcine insulin in the solution (biphasic insulin only), and their zinc-ion content. The crystalline part of biphasic insulin contains only the amount of zinc ions (4 Zn/hexamer) necessary for crystallization, and essentially all Zn^{2+} is structurally bound in the crystals. In contrast, the IZS preparations contain a large surplus of zinc ions, of which only approximately 50% are bound to the crystals. As illustrated in Fig. 8 the presence of free zinc ions rather than pH seems to be crucial for the formation of the split product.

Effect of Temperature

The temperature dependence of the different hydrolysis reactions is shown in Table VI, in which the coefficient Q_{10} is calculated for different temperature intervals. An increasing effect of temperature on the rate of B3 transformation by raising the temperature by 10°C can be observed, especially for the N2 formulation. The coefficients for the B3 transformation are approximately 3 (4–25°C) for most formulations, whereas the corresponding temperature coefficients for the

Table V. Initial Rate Constants of Formation of Desamido and Split Products in Insulin Zinc Suspensions, Crystalline[a]

Insulin species	Desamido-(B3)-insulin, 25°C	Split-(A8–A9)-product		
		4°C	15°C	25°C
Human	1.0			0.4
	(0.04, n = 8)			(0.1, n = 5)
Porcine	0.2	0.008	0.14	1.0
	(0.01, n = 5)	(0.001, n = 10)	(0.02, n = 8)	(0.1, n = 10)
Bovine	<0.02	0.05	0.52	5.9
		(0.01, n = 9)	(0.04, n = 9)	(0.2, n = 6)

[a] The rate data ($k \times 10^2$/month $\pm$ SE) are calculated from the initial linear part of the curves; see Fig. 6.

formation of the split product in porcine and bovine IZS cryst. formulations are approximately three times higher.

Manufacturer

There seem to be no major differences among four manufacturers with respect to the formation of the isoAsp[B3] hydrolysis product in different preparations or formation of the A8–A9 split product in the IZS mixed type of preparation (Table VII).

Other Degradation Products

When using disc electrophoresis other possible insulin transformation products were below the detection limit (approximately 0.2% by visual inspection), but by using the more sensitive two-step HPLC method (with initial removal of di- and polymerization products), supplemental distinct

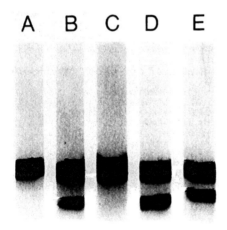

A B C D E

Fig. 8. Gel electrophoresis (performed as disc electrophoresis) of different formulations of bovine insulin zinc suspensions, crystalline (40 IU/ml), after storage of the preparations for 2 months at 37°C. (A) Containing 12 μg Zn^{2+} ml, corresponding to the amount of zinc structurally bound to the insulin (4 zinc atoms/hexamer of insulin), pH 7.0; (B) 83 μg Zn^{2+}/ml, pH 7.0; (C) 12 μg Zn^{2+}/ml, pH 7.5; (D) 83 μg Zn^{2+}/ml, pH 7.5; (E) for comparison, porcine insulin containing 10% monodesamido-(A21)-insulin.

peaks in the chromatogram were observed to increase with time. However, these additional transformation products with approximately the same molecular weight as insulin are distributed over 10–15 peaks in the chromatogram.

Calculation of the total sum of all these additional insulin transformation products (excluding di- and polymerization products; see the following paper) detectable by RP-HPLC reveals that ≤0.3% (versus 1–2% of the B3 transformation product) is formed per month at 25°C, with a tendency to slightly higher values for regular N2 than for N1.

DISCUSSION

This study demonstrates the following.

(1) Deamidation of insulin occurs in neutral solution but the rate of formation is reduced by one order of magnitude compared to the rate of deamidation at residue A21 in acid formulations.

(2) In neutral solutions and suspensions deamidation takes place almost exclusively at residue Asn[B3] and leads to a mixture of aspartyl and isoaspartyl derivatives.

(3) The rate of hydrolysis is independent of the concentration (strength) and, in most cases, the species of insulin (human, porcine, or bovine) but is strongly influenced by the composition and formulation of the preparations.

(4) The ratio at which the isoAsp[B3] and Asp[B3] derivatives are formed is independent of time and temperature but varies with the formulation. In neutral solution the formation of the isoAsp derivative dominates relative to the Asp derivative, whereas the transformation of insulin in suspension leads mainly to formation of the Asp[B3] derivative.

(5) In certain crystalline insulin suspensions cleavage of the peptide bond A8–A9 can be observed. This hydrolytic cleavage of the A chain takes place only in suspensions containing rhombohedral crystals in addition to a relatively high Zn^{2+} content (>4 Zn/hexamer). Rate of formation of the A8–A9 split product is species dependent (bovine > porcine > human insulin).

Deamidation Reactions

Site and Mechanism

Deamidation of glutaminyl and asparaginyl residues in peptides and proteins has been extensively studied and reviewed by Robinson and Rudd (12), who concluded that the rate of deamidation is dependent upon the primary sequence, secondary and tertiary structure, temperature, pH, ion strength, and special intermolecular interactions. They

Table VI. Effect of Temperature on the Rate of Hydrolysis of Insulin in Neutral Formulations[a]

| | Temperature interval (°C) | | | | | |
| | B3 deamidation | | | | | A8–A9 cleavage |
Preparation	4–15	15–25	4–25	25–37	37–45	4–25
Regular N1	3.2	3.2	3.2	5.2	2.4	
Regular N2	2.6	3.3	2.9	3.7	3.7	
IZS, amorphous			3.3			
IZS, crystalline						
Bovine						9.7
Porcine			3.1			10.0
Isophane (NPH)			1.4			
Biphasic			3.1			

[a] The figures, calculated from data for the individual products in Tables III–V, are the temperature coefficient Q_{10}, i.e., the increase in rate of reaction when the temperature increases 10°C in the temperature interval indicated.

also showed that asparaginyl residues are much more prone to deamidation than glutaminyl residues.

Insulin deamidates rapidly in acid formulations due to hydrolysis at residue Asn^{A21} (3). The particular lability of the A21 amide is due to its position as a C-terminal residue, where deamidation is catalyzed by the terminal uncharged carboxyl group (18,19).

A mechanism for deamidation at neutral pH of asparaginyl residues involving formation of a cyclic succinimide intermediate followed by nucleophilic attack by hydroxide ion was proposed by Bornstein and Balian (20). This process leads to the formation of a mixture of peptides in which the polypeptide backbone is attached via an alpha-carboxyl linkage (Asp) or via a beta-carboxyl linkage (isoAsp). Strong evidence for this pathway as the dominating mechanism for deamidation in peptides and proteins has been obtained in studies of synthetic model peptides (13,17,21,22) and of proteins (11,23–25). The succinimide formation has been shown to be dependent on the charge and size of the side chain on the adjacent carboxyl-site residue (12,13) but recent investigations have emphasized the role of tertiary structure and its influence on the conformational restraints on imide formation (17,19,22,26).

The rate-determining step in the deamidation reaction

via the cyclic imide is the formation of the intermediate succinimide, which is a much slower process than the subsequent hydrolysis into Asp and isoAsp peptides (13,24).

Deamidation at Residue Asn^{B3}

The transformation of insulin in neutral medium into two B3 derivatives probably also involves the formation of a cyclic imide intermediate which hydrolyzes under retention of either a normal peptide linkage corresponding to simple deamidation or a beta-carboxyl linkage (isopeptide).

For neutral solutions as well as suspensions the lowest rates of deamidation are seen when the preparations contain phenol (regular N2 and NPH, respectively). This apparent effect of phenol is consistent with the fact that the B1–B8 α-helix induced by phenol (27,28) reduces the flexibility around the B3 residue and thereby the possibilities for imide formation. The two neutral solutions differ not only with respect to rate of deamidation but also in their time courses of degradation. Regular N2, especially at the lower temperatures, exhibits a more linear course than regular N1, in which the rate of degradation at all temperatures decreases with time (negative b values at all temperatures). In the latter preparation hydrolysis of methylparaben into p-hydroxyben-

Table VII. Influence of the Brand of Insulin on Deamidation and Split Product Formation

| Brand[a] | Storage temperature (°C) | Formation of isoAsp[B3] derivative in human insulin preparations (% per month) | | | Formation of split product in IZS, mixed (bovine crystals) (% per week) |
		Regular N2	NPH	IZS, cryst.	
A	25	0.77	0.20	0.32	
	37	2.1	0.6	1.3	
	45				2.0
B	25	0.56	0.23		
	37	1.8	1.0		
C	25	0.63	0.12		
	37	2.0	0.6		
D	25	0.62	0.15	0.29	
	37	1.9	0.7	0.9	
	45				2.0

[a] One or two batches of each brand were analyzed by HPLC.

zoic acid leads to a fall in pH during storage (8), whereas a more constant pH applies to regular N2. Therefore the decreasing B3 deamidation with falling pH in the range 6.8 to 7.6 (data not shown) may account for the different time courses in deamidation of the two neutral solutions.

The insulins of different animal species have identical primary structure at the B-chain N terminal, and it is therefore not surprising that they exhibit the same tendency to deamidation. One exception are the preparations in which the parallel occurring and species-dependent cleavage of the A-chain probably causes an overall change in the flexibility of the molecule.

Human insulin was proposed to be more susceptible to chemical transformation, including deamidation, than bovine insulin (29), but this observation is flawed by the fact that the two neutral preparations also varied with respect to formulation and initial purity.

The total hydrolytic transformation at Asn^{B3} occurs to the same extent in neutral medium containing identical auxiliary substances (NaCl and methylparaben) regardless of whether insulin is in the amorphous state (IZS, amorph.) or in solution (regular N1), indicating similar conformational flexibility and propensity to imide formation at B3. In contrast, when the insulin in suspension is in the crystalline rather than the amorphous state, the transformation at B3 is considerably reduced (Table IV). In the amorphous suspension insulin is precipitated with the individual insulin hexamers loosely packed together in an unordered way, probably with zinc ions binding them together, whereas in the rhombohedral crystals (IZS type of preparation) the hexamers are closely packed, with many direct contacts between the individual hexamers (30). These constraints on the tertiary structure reduce the possibilities for the large movement of the B-chain N terminal necessary for the peptide bond nitrogen atom to approach the B3 side-chain carbonyl carbon in order to form the succinimide ring (23). In the monoclinic NPH crystals the hexamers are more loosely packed, but the phenol content of this formulation induces helix formation at B1–B8, which adds to the conformational stability in this region of the molecule. Thus, the structural restraints put on the insulin molecule when in the crystalline form account for the slow rate of deamidation in the crystalline formulations. In comparison, in the formulations with insulin in the amorphous or dissolved form, allowing more conformational flexibility in the molecule, imide formation at B3 is facilitated, leading to a faster rate of deamidation. These results strongly support the theory that tertiary structure is the main determinant for protein deamidation (17,19,22,26).

Ratio of IsoAsp/Asp Derivatives

The ratios of B3 isomerized to B3 normal peptide observed in the neutral solutions are lower than that seen in deamidation of oligopeptides (13,17) but similar to the value seen in deamidation of α-crystalline subunits (24). The reason for such reduced values might be an additional deamidation pathway via direct solvent hydrolysis of the side-chain amide. However, Meinwald et al. (21), in studies on deamidation of asparaginyl-glycyl model peptides, were not able to detect any direct side-chain hydrolysis of the primary amide. The independence of the ratios on time and temperature also indicates that all deamidation proceeds via the imide. It would also be difficult to understand why any direct hydrolysis of the amide in B3 in neutral solution would not occur at the other two Asn residues in insulin. Therefore the reduced ratio is more likely explained by the lower accessibility to hydrolysis of the peptide linkage (isoaspartyl formation) as compared to the other hydrolyzable bond in the imide when this is part of a large peptide with more fixed tertiary structure.

The phenol-containing regular N2 gives a lower isoAsp/ Asp ratio than regular N1 with methylparaben as preservative. Thus, the helix formation induced by phenol not only reduces the possibilities for imide formation but also apparently decreases the accessibility of the main chain for hydrolysis relative to the side-chain part of the imide.

Whereas formation of the isoAsp derivative dominates in solution, the Asp derivative is the main hydrolytic product when insulin is in suspension. This is probably due to further reduced accessibility of the carbonyl carbon in the peptide linkage for nucleophilic attack by water (or OH^-) when insulin is in the amorphous or crystalline phase rather than in solution. In that respect the amorphous state is not different from the crystalline state of insulin, as similar ratios of isoAsp/Asp can be observed (Table IV).

The trend toward lower isoAsp/Asp ratios with more stabilized structures of the molecule (effect of phenol and crystallization) indicates that tertiary structure is governing not only imide formation but also the subsequent hydrolysis reactions.

Electrophoretic Mobility of the Deamidation Products

An interesting and peculiar phenomenon in relation to the $isoAsp^{B3}$ insulin derivatives from different species of insulin is their electrophoretic mobilities on the disc gel (Fig. 3). In the electrophoresis buffer (pH 8) the Asp and the isoAsp derivatives both carry a full extra negative charge relative to insulin. Nonetheless, these two derivatives are clearly separated on the disc gel when they are derived from porcine and human insulin, with the isoAsp derivatives moving approx. 30% (relative to insulin) ahead of the other derivative, whereas the two derivatives formed from bovine insulin have the same mobility (that bovine insulin actually is hydrolyzed into the same two derivatives formed at the same ratio has been proven in ion-exchange experiments). As disc gel electrophoresis separates according to charge and also to molecular size, its efficacy in separating the porcine and human derivatives could be explained by the $isoAsp^{B3}$ insulin molecule being slightly smaller in size (more folded tertiary structure). The differences in primary structure (A8 and A10 residues) are located not too far from the B3 residue in the tertiary structure. Therefore, the substitution of A8 Ala in bovine insulin with Thr in human and porcine insulin may, in combination with the conformational changes induced in the main chain (an extra carbon atom) by the isomerization of B3, creates possibilities for hydrogen bonding between the side chain of Thr A8 and the B-chain N-terminal residues. This could result in a more folded and compact molecule in the isoAsp derivatives of human and porcine insulin than in that of bovine insulin.

Hydrolytic Cleavage of the Peptide Bond A8–A9

The cleavage of the peptide bond between residue A8 (Ala in bovine and Thr in porcine and human insulin) and residue A9 (Ser in all three species) is quite unusual, and a similar spontaneous reaction dependent on the presence of higher concentrations of zinc ions has apparently not been described for other nonenzyme proteins. The crucial role played by the availability of free zinc ions (Fig. 8) explains why formation of the split product cannot be detected in the otherwise identical rhombohedral crystals in the biphasic formulation.

The peptide bond involving the amino group of Ser is known to be labile and susceptible to hydrolysis via N–O acyl rearrangement but the intermediate peptidyl shift requires strong acidic conditions. The cleavage is most likely due to an autoproteolytic, metalloproteinase-mediated cleavage by the adjacent hexamer in the stacking of hexamers in the rhombohedral crystal. The key element for enzyme activity, a Glu carboxylate group, is available from the adjacent hexamer, and a zinc ion, supposed to be coordinated to one Glu and two His in the Michaelis complex (31), is available from the medium. This autocatalytic theory is supported by the insulin species variation in the split product formation. Thus bovine insulin with the fastest formation actually has the closest interactions between hexamers in this part of the crystal. The different rate of formation of the split product when comparing bovine insulin with human and porcine insulin can also be accounted for by primary structure differences (A8 Ala and Thr, respectively). The slightly faster formation in porcine relative to human crystals can be explained only by differences in the three-dimensional packing of the hexamers.

The split product formation proceeds initially relatively rapidly, whereafter it slows down (Fig. 6) and eventually stops. As its formation decreased substantially with falling pH (data not shown), this time course is probably caused by the decrease in pH during storage of the IZS preparations (8).

Effect of Temperature

The relatively large temperature effect observed for the B3 deamidation reaction (Table VI), especially around 30°C, most likely reflects the increase in conformational freedom at the deamidating B3 residue with increasing temperature. Because formation of the succinimide ring is rate determining in the transformation reaction (13), the overall reaction is facilitated when higher temperatures increase the possibility for the main-chain and side-chain groups to assume the conformation necessary for succinimide formation. Thus, stereochemical factors also govern the effect of temperature on the deamidation of Asn[B3]. The much higher temperature effect seen for formation of the split product probably indicates the need for weakening of the conformational interactions within the hexamer before the approach between hexamers can be sufficiently close for the catalytic reaction to take place.

Impact on the Quality of the Preparations

The hydrolytic reactions occurring during storage of in-sulin preparations are quantitatively predominant and cause transformation of substantially larger amounts of insulin than the parallel occurring di- and polymerization reactions (10). The molecular changes induced by deamidation are relatively small, although the isoAsp formation, in addition to changing the uncharged Asn residue into a charged Asp group, also introduces an extra carbon atom into the peptide backbone. This may cause more extensive structural changes. However, the deamidation products have essentially the same in vivo biological potency as the intact molecule (8), and also the immunogenicity in rabbit experiments has been found not to differ from that of the parent insulin (8,9).

The rate-determining step in the deamidation reaction is the formation of the cyclic imide (13,21). Geiger and Clarke (13) found the rate of imide formation in an asparaginyl hexapeptide approximately 40 times slower than the subsequent hydrolysis reaction and calculated the steady-state concentration of the succinimide intermediate to be about 0.2%. Therefore accumulation of the insulin B3 succinimide during storage is likely to be insignificant compared with the end products.

The cleavage of the peptide backbone of the A chain between position A8 and position A9 represents a much more dramatic change and probably induces major alterations in the three-dimensional structure of the molecule. The cleavage is close to two disulfide bridges (A6–A11 and A7–B7), one of which connects the two separated A-chain peptides (A1–A8 and A9–A21) in the split product. Together these disulfide bridges will probably be able to keep the molecule in its folded state and maintain most of the overall tertiary structure, but the much larger retention on the HPLC column (Fig. 2) indicates exposure of some of the hydrophobic core to the surface of the molecule. In accordance, the biological in vivo potency of the split product is only about 2% of that of the parent hormone (15). The relatively low biological stability of the preparations containing rhombohedral crystals in combination with surplus zinc ions (IZS cryst. and IZS mixed), especially at higher storage temperatures (2,8), can essentially be accounted for by the split product formation. When stored as recommended (temperature interval, 2–8°C), the fall in potency during shelf life would, however, be less than 5% for the bovine IZS cryst. preparation. Assuming the same temperature coefficient Q_{10} for human as for porcine split product formation, the fall in potency in the human IZS cryst. preparation due to split product formation is calculated to be about 1% after 2 years at 15°C.

Animal insulins vary mainly in primary structure within the A-chain loop (A8 to A10) and these mutations are known to have a great impact on the immunogenicity of the insulin (32). Therefore it could be expected that the molecular change induced by the cleavage of the backbone in the split product would also lead to increased immunogenicity. However, the porcine split product showed the same low immunogenicity in rabbit experiments as the intact parent molecule (15). Insulin preparations formulated with the same species of insulin are generally seen to induce more antibody formation when formulated as a protracted rather than a rapid-acting preparation (33,34). It is, therefore, still an open question whether this enhanced immunogenicity is due primarily to the prolonged stay of insulin in subcutis or to the content of insulin transformation products such as the split product and covalent insulin dimers (35).

ACKNOWLEDGMENTS

The authors wish to acknowledge the skillful technical assistance of Lene Grønlund Andersen, Lene Bramsen, Liselotte Fensby, Lise Frank, Jessie Frederiksen, Birgit Jensen, Lone Jørgensen, Anne-Marie Kolstrup, Eva Bøg Kristensen, Jette Laulund, Harriet Markussen, and Birgit Dræby Spon. We are grateful to Professor Guy Dodson, University of York, England, for helpful discussions and to Klaus Jørgensen, Novo Research Institute, and Professor Francis C. Szoka, Jr., University of California, San Francisco, for critically reading the manuscript and for valuable comments. We also thank Kathleen Larsen for help with preparing the manuscript.

REFERENCES

1. W. O. Storvick and H. J. Henry. Effect of storage temperature on stability of commercial insulin preparations. *Diabetes* 17:499–502 (1968).
2. M. Pingel and A. Vølund. Stability of insulin preparations. *Diabetes* 21:805–813 (1972).
3. F. Sundby. Separation and characterization of acid-induced insulin transformation products by paper electrophoresis in 7 M urea. *J. Biol. Chem.* 237:3406–3411 (1962).
4. L. I. Slobin and F. H. Carpenter. The labile amide in insulin: Preparation of desalanine-desamido-insulin. *Biochemistry* 2:22–28 (1963).
5. B. V. Fisher and P. B. Porter. Stability of bovine insulin. *J. Pharm. Pharmacol.* 33:203–206 (1981).
6. R. L. Jackson, W. O. Storvick, C. S. Hollinden, L. E. Stroeh, and J. G. Stilz. Neutral regular insulin. *Diabetes* 21:235–245 (1972).
7. J. Schlichtkrull, M. Pingel, L. G. Heding, J. Brange, and K. H. Jørgensen. Insulin preparations with prolonged effect. In A. Hasselblatt and F. von Bruchhausen (eds.), *Handbook of Experimental Pharmacology, New Series, Vol. XXXII/2*, Springer-Verlag, Berlin, Heidelberg, New York, 1975, pp. 729–777.
8. J. Brange, B. Skelbaek-Pedersen, L. Langkjaer, U. Damgaard, H. Ege, S. Havelund, L. G. Heding, K. H. Jørgensen, J. Lykkeberg, J. Markussen, M. Pingel, and E. Rasmussen. *Galenics of Insulin: The Physico-chemical and Pharmaceutical Aspects of Insulin and Insulin Preparations*, Springer-Verlag, Berlin, Heidelberg, New York, London, Paris, Tokyo, 1987.
9. J. Schlichtkrull, J. Brange, A. H. Christiansen, O. Hallund, L. G. Heding, K. H. Jørgensen, S. M. Rasmussen, E. Sørensen, and A. Vølund. Monocomponent insulin and its clinical implications. *Horm. Metab. Res. (Suppl. Ser.)* 5:134–143 (1974).
10. J. Brange, S. Havelund, and P. Hougaard. Chemical stability of insulin. 2. Formation of higher molecular weight transformation products during storage of pharmaceutical preparations. *Pharm. Res.* 9:727–734 (1992).
11. M. C. Manning, K. Patel, and R. T. Borchardt. Stability of protein pharmaceuticals. *Pharm. Res.* 6:903–918 (1989).
12. A. B. Robinson and C. J. Rudd. Deamidation of glutaminyl and asparaginyl residues in peptides and proteins. *Current Topics in Cellular Regulation, Vol. 8*, Academic Press, New York, 1974, pp. 247–295.
13. T. Geiger and S. Clarke. Deamidation, isomerization, and racemization at asparaginyl and aspartyl residues in peptides. Succinimide-linked reactions that contribute to protein degradation. *J. Biol. Chem.* 262:785–794 (1987).
14. J. Brange, L. Langkjær, S. Havelund, and E. Sørensen. Chem-

ical stability of insulin: Neutral insulin solutions. *Diabetologia* 25:193 (1983) (abstr).
15. J. Brange, L. Langkjær, S. Havelund, and E. Sørensen. Chemical stability of insulin: Formation of desamidido insulins and other hydrolytic products in intermediate- and long-acting insulin preparations. *Diabetes Res. Clin. Pract. Suppl.* 1:67 (1985) (abstr).
16. J. Brange, S. Havelund, E. Hommel, E. Sørensen, and C. Kühl. Neutral insulin solutions physically stabilized by addition of Zn^{2+}. *Diabet. Med.* 3:532–536 (1986).
17. R. Lura and V. Schirch. Role of peptide conformation in the rate and mechanism of deamidation of asparaginyl residues. *Biochemistry* 27:7671–7677 (1988).
18. S. J. Leach and H. Lindley. The kinetics of hydrolysis of the amide group in proteins and peptides. Part 2. Acid hydrolysis of glycyl- and l-leucyl-l-asparagine. *Trans. Faraday Soc.* 49:921–925 (1953).
19. H. T. Wright. Sequence and structure determinants of the nonenzymatic deamidation of asparagin and glutamine residues in proteins. *Protein Eng.* 4:283–294 (1991).
20. P. Bornstein and G. Balian. Cleavage at Asn-Gly bonds with hydroxylamine. *Methods Enzymol.* 47:132–145 (1977).
21. Y. C. Meinwald, E. R. Stimson, and H. A. Scheraga. Deamidation of the asparaginyl-glycyl sequence. *Int. J. Peptide Protein Res.* 28:79–84 (1986).
22. R. C. Stephenson and S. Clarke. Succinimide formation from aspartyl and asparaginyl peptides as a model for the spontaneous degradation of proteins. *J. Biol. Chem.* 264:6164–6170 (1989).
23. S. Clarke. Propensity for spontaneous succinimide formation from aspartyl and asparaginyl residues in cellular proteins. *Int. J. Peptide Protein Res.* 30:808–821 (1987).
24. C. E. M. Voorter, W. A. de Haard-Hoekman, P. J. M. van den Oetelaar, H. Bloemendal, and W. W. de Jong. Spontaneous peptide bond cleavage in aging α-crystallin through a succinimide intermediate. *J. Biol. Chem.* 263:19020–19023 (1988).
25. N. P. Bhatt, K. Patel, and R. T. Borchardt. Chemical pathways of peptide degradation. I. Deamidation of adrenocorticotropic hormone. *Pharm. Res.* 7:593–599 (1990).
26. A. A. Kossiakoff. Tertiary structure is a principal determinant to protein deamidation. *Science* 240:191–194 (1988).
27. A. Wollmer, B. Rannefeld, B. R. Johansen, K. R. Hejnaes, P. Balschmidt, and F. B. Hansen. Phenol-promoted structural transformation of insulin in solution. *Biol. Chem. Hoppe-Seyler* 368:903–911 (1987).
28. U. Derewenda, Z. Derewenda, E. J. Dodson, G. G. Dodson, C. D. Reynolds, G. D. Smith, C. Sparks, and D. Swenson. Phenol stabilizes more helix in a new symmetrical zinc insulin hexamer. *Nature* 338:594–596 (1989).
29. R. Gregory, S. Edwards, and N. A. Yateman. Demonstration of insulin transformation products in insulin vials by high-performance liquid chromatography. *Diabetes Care* 14:42–48 (1991).
30. E. N. Baker, T. L. Blundell, J. F. Cutfield, S. M. Cutfield, E. J. Dodson, G. G. Dodson, D. M. C. Hodgkin, R. E. Hubbard, N. W. Isaacs, C. D. Reynolds, K. Sakabe, N. Sakabe, and N. M. Vijayan. The structure of 2Zn pig insulin crystals at 1.5 Å resolution. *Phil. Trans. R. Soc.* 319:369–456 (1988).
31. S. Toma, S. Campagnoli, E. De Gregoriis, R. Gianna, I. Margarit, M. Zamai, and G. Grandi. Effect of Glu-143 and His-231 substitutions on the catalytic activity and secretion of bacillus subtilis neutral protease. *Protein Eng.* 2:359–364 (1989).
32. W. G. Reeves. Immunogenicity of insulin of various origins. *Neth. J. Med.* 28 (Suppl 1):43–46 (1985).
33. S. Fankhauser. Neuere Aspekte der Insulintherapie. *Schweiz Med. Wochenschr.* 99:414–420 (1969).
34. N. S. Fineberg, S. E. Fineberg, R. J. Mahler, and L. G. Linarelli. Is regular human insulin less immunogenic than repository? *Diabetes* 35 (Suppl 1):91A (1986) (abstr).
35. D. C. Robbins, S. M. Cooper, S. E. Fineberg, and P. M. Mead. Antibodies to covalent aggregates of insulin in blood of insulin-using diabetic patients. *Diabetes* 36:838–841 (1987).

Reproduced from *Pharmaceutical Research*, 9(6):727–734, 1992.

Chemical Stability of Insulin.
2. Formation of Higher Molecular Weight Transformation Products During Storage of Pharmaceutical Preparations

Jens Brange,[1,2] Svend Havelund,[1] and
Philip Hougaard[1]

Received August 22, 1991; accepted December 22, 1991

Formation of covalent, higher molecular weight transformation (HMWT) products during storage of insulin preparations at 4–45°C was studied by size exclusion chromatography. The main products are covalent insulin dimers (CID), but in protamine-containing preparations the concurrent formation of covalent insulin–protamine (CIP) products takes place. At temperatures ≥25°C parallel or consecutive formation of covalent oligo- and polymers can also be observed. Rate of HMWT is only slightly influenced by species of insulin but varies with composition and formulation, and for isophane (NPH) preparations, also with the strength of preparation. Temperature has a pronounced effect on CID, CIP, and, especially, covalent oligo- and polymer formation. The CIDs are apparently formed between molecules within the hexameric unit common for all types of preparations and rate of formation is generally faster in glycerol-containing preparations. Compared with insulin hydrolysis reactions (see the preceding paper), HMWT is one order of magnitude slower, except for NPH preparations.

KEY WORDS: insulin; insulin preparation; chemical stability; covalent dimerization; polymerization; covalent insulin protamine.

INTRODUCTION

In the preceding paper (1) the chemical degradation of insulin in pharmaceutical formulations was studied with respect to formation of hydrolytic degradation products. However, insulin in preparations has also been found to be chemically transformed by formation of insulin di- and polymerization products (2–5).

Steiner and co-workers were the first to show the presence of a ("nonconvertible") insulin dimer in insulin crystals (6) and suggested that it was an artifact associated with commercial production (7). Similar covalent dimers have been isolated by Helbig (8) as a heterogeneous mixture of different insulin derivatives, in some of which the N-terminal amino groups from one insulin molecule had reacted with the A21 amido group from another molecule. Partial dimerization of insulin at pH 7 as a result of disulfide exchange was reported by Csorba *et al.* (9). The potential sites for formation of such

[1] Novo Research Institute, Novo Alle, DK-2880 Bagsvaerd, Denmark.

[2] To whom correspondence should be addressed at Novo Research Institute, Novo Alle, DK-2880 Bagsvaerd, Denmark.

insulin transamidation (intermolecular aminolysis) and disulfide exchange products are illustrated in Fig. 1.

We report in this communication the formation of covalent, higher molecular weight transformation (HMWT) products during storage of insulin preparations of different types and formulations, as revealed by the appearance of peaks eluting in front of the insulin peak when analyzed by size exclusion chromatography (SEC). Preliminary accounts have been published in abstract form (3,4) and in excerpt (5). For detailed information about the different types of insulin preparations studied, reference is made to the preceding paper (1).

MATERIALS AND METHODS

Materials

Insulins and chemicals used and the preparation of the different formulations were described in the preceding article, in which also a survey of the different preparations and their content of auxiliary substances were included (Ref. 1, Tables I and II). The majority of batches was from the production line of Novo Industri A/S, but batches produced on a smaller scale in the laboratory were also studied. The insulin preparations including samples from other manufacturers were handled as described earlier (1).

Methods

Isolation and Storage of Samples. Dissolved insulin was isolated by zinc precipitation and subsequent centrifugation as described earlier (1). Due to the requirements of low ion strength mentioned below, the precipitate was washed with 20 μl of 1 mM zinc acetate/mg of insulin precipitate. Insulin in suspensions was isolated by centrifugation and washed as described above. Samples were stored, without drying, in the deep freeze (-20°C) until analysis.

Analytical Procedures. Samples were analyzed for content of HMWT products either by conventional size exclusion chromatography (CSEC) or by high-performance size exclusion chromatography (HPSEC). CSEC was performed on columns (25 × 400 mm) of Bio-Gel P 30, 100–200 mesh (Bio-Rad Laboratories) equilibrated for at least 20 hr with 1 M acetic acid in order to ensure the lowest possible baseline readings. Separation efficiency of each column packing was checked by running a standard impure insulin sample (once-crystallized porcine insulin) and columns were repacked after every 10 runs. Insulin samples (10–100 mg of insulin depending on the expected content of HMWT products) were dissolved in 2 M acetic acid and applied on the column in a total volume not exceeding 1.5 ml. It was found necessary to keep the ion strength of the applied sample as low as possible in order to avoid artificial splitting of the insulin peak into two peaks. In cases of voluminous insulin samples (amorphously precipitated insulin) from preparations made isotonic with NaCl, the salt content in the supernatant was reduced by washing with 1 mM zinc acetate and centrifugation. Elution with 1 M acetic acid was performed at ambient temperature at a rate of 3 cm/hr and 1.5-ml fractions were

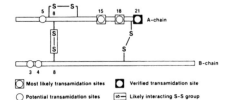

Fig. 1. A schematic illustration of potential sites involved in covalent di- and polymerization of insulin.

collected. Insulin and HMWT products were detected as the area under the curve by measuring absorbance at 276 nm. As protamine has no absorbance at this wavelength, the measured amount of CIP is not a weight fraction but accounts only for the fraction of chemically transformed insulin. Using the procedure described the detection limit for HMWT products was found to be 0.05–0.1% and reproducibility was approx. ±3% for estimation of CID content above 1% (coefficient of variation = 0.033, $n = 7$) and ±9% for values below 1% (CV = 0.094, $n = 6$). For a covalent polymer content of about 2%, the reproducibility was ±6% (CV = 0.056, $n = 5$).

HPSEC was performed on a Waters I-125 column (7.8 × 300 mm) using an eluent with 2.5 M acetic acid, 4 mM l-arginine, and 4% (v/v) acetonitrile. Elution was performed at ambient temperature at a rate of 1 ml/min and insulin and HMWT products were detected by their absorbance at 280 nm. The reproducibility of this method was found to be similar to that of the CSEC method.

Data Analysis. The experimental data were analyzed by least-squares polynomial regression analysis including a linear and a quadratic term:

$$D = at + bt^2$$

where D is the fraction of transformed insulin as percentage of total and t is time as months. In the cases where coefficient b is not significantly different from zero, using a statistical significance level of 0.05, the quadratic term is excluded. Results are generally quoted as the initial rate constant, i.e., a, and its standard error, supplemented with b when it is significant. Significance testing was performed by standard F tests.

RESULTS

Covalent insulin dimer (CID) products are formed in all types of insulin formulations during storage of the preparations. In the preparations formulated with protamine an extra peak eluting in front of the peak containing the CID products can be observed at all storage temperatures. This peak which has been shown to contain reaction products of insulin linked covalently to protamine (10) is subsequently referred to as covalent insulin protamine (CIP). At higher storage temperatures (≥25°C) additional formation of covalent insulin polymerization products can be observed in all preparations. Figures 2 and 3 illustrate the diversity in the time

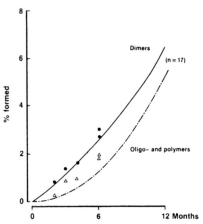

Fig. 2. Time courses of formation of dimers (——) and oligo- and polymers (– · – · – ·) during storage of regular N1 porcine insulin at 37°C. The lines represent the best fits of data ($n = 17$) on preparations of U 40 strength. Additional data on formation of covalent dimers (●) and oligo- and polymers (△) in preparations of U 100 strength reveal a tendency to increased formation of covalent oligo- and polymers with increasing strength of insulin.

courses of formation of the HMWT products in different types of pharmaceutical insulin preparations.

Rate Data

Rate data for the different types of preparation with respect to the total formation of HMWT products are shown in Tables I–III. Except for the protamine-containing prepa-

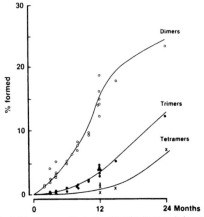

Fig. 3. Time courses of formation of insulin oligomers during storage of insulin zinc suspension, crystalline (bovine or porcine), at 37°C.

Table I. Total HMWT Product Formation in Protamine-Containing Preparations[a]

Preparation	Species[b]	Strength	Temperature (°C) 4	15	25	37	45
NPH	Bovine	U 100	3.1 ± 0.7 (n = 8) n.s.	6.6 ± 1.1 (n = 8) P < 0.05	22.1 ± 1.4 (n = 14) P < 0.001	116 ± 33 (n = 5) P < 0.05	
	P and H	U 100	4.0 ± 0.5 (n = 23) n.s.	9.7 ± 0.9 (n = 17) P < 0.001	27.8 ± 1.0 (n = 34) P < 0.001	160 ± 5 (n = 20) P < 0.05	462 ± 27 b = −92[c] (n = 9) P < 0.001
	P and H	U 40	5.0 ± 0.4 (n = 31) n.s.	18.9 ± 1.6 (n = 24) P < 0.01	53.7 ± 3.0 b = −0.6 (n = 46) P < 0.001	271 ± 17 b = −19 (n = 31)	773 ± 48 b = −178 (n = 6)
	P	U 80	3.8 ± 0.8 (n = 10)	14.0 ± 1.3 (n = 11)	27.0 ± 2.7 (n = 10)		
PZI	P	U 40	6.2 ± 0.8 (n = 11)	16.3 ± 0.5 (n = 7)	80 ± 9 (n = 8)	1180 ± 80 b = −98 (n = 4)	

[a] Figures are the apparent first-order rate constants ($\times 10^4$ month^{-1}) ± SE.
[b] P, porcine; H, human.
[c] b values ($\times 10^4$), the coefficient to the quadratic term, are given when the polynomial expression gives the best fit of the time course.

rations, the CID fraction is the only kind of HMWT product formed at the lower storage temperatures (4–15°C). Data for the parallel formation of CID and CIP products during storage of NPH at several temperatures are listed in Table IV. At the higher storage temperatures (25–45°C) additional formation of products with a MW higher than the CID occurs in some of the preparations (Table V).

Effect of Concentration and Species of Insulin

For most preparations there is no major influence of the insulin concentration on the formation of CID. In contrast, increasing the concentration of insulin in neutral solution tends to increase the rate of formation of covalent oligo- and polymers at the higher storage temperatures (Fig. 2 and Table VI). The NPH formulation is the only type of preparation in which the strength of insulin has a highly significant effect on the formation of HMWT products including CID as well as CIP (Table I and IV).

There is no overall tendency that one particular species of insulin is more stable than another. Thus bovine insulin is the most stable species of insulin in the NPH formulation but exhibits the fastest rate of transformation when used in the regular N1 formulation. Generally human and porcine insulin exhibit the same rate of HMWT product formation, and only in the preparations containing rhombohedral crystals [insulin zinc suspensions (IZS), crystalline and mixed] is porcine insulin significantly more stable than human insulin.

Effect of Composition and Formulation

In neutral solution formation of HMWT products is 40–160% higher in regular N2 (with phenol + glycerol) compared to regular N1 (with methylparaben + NaCl) (Table III). In the protamine-containing preparations, neutral protamine Hagedorn (NPH; crystalline suspension) and protamine zinc insulin (PZI; amorphous suspension), formation of HMWT products is comparable at the lower temperatures, but at 25 and 37°C the PZI formulation is becoming increasingly more unstable than the crystalline NPH preparation (Table I). The same tendency to inferior stability of amorphously precipitated insulin at the higher storage temperatures, when compared with insulin in crystalline suspension, can be observed for the IZS type of preparation (Table II).

Manufacturer

Comparison of human insulin preparations from four manufacturers revealed that the rate of formation of HMWT products in neutral solutions can vary up to 100% between different manufacturers, whereas only small differences are seen within NPH preparations of the same strength (Fig. 4).

DISCUSSION

The present study demonstrates the following.

(1) Intermolecular chemical reactions occur in all pharmaceutical insulin formulations but at rates which are generally much slower than those observed for hydrolytic reactions (1).

(2) CID are the main products formed in most preparations, but in protamine-containing preparations the concurrent formation of covalent insulin–protamine reaction products takes place at all storage temperatures.

(3) At storage temperatures ≥25°C parallel or consecutive reactions are seen in most types of preparations, resulting in the formation of covalent insulin oligo- and polymers.

Table II. Total HMWT Product Formation in Insulin Zinc Suspensions (IZS Types of Preparations)[a]

Table II. Total HMWT Product Formation in Insulin Zinc Suspensions (IZS Types of Preparations)[a]

Preparation	Species[b]	Strength	Temperature (°C) 4	15	25	37	45
IZS, amorph.	P	U 40, 80	0.28 ± 0.06 (n = 12)	1.2 ± 0.1 (n = 15)	7.9 ± 0.3 (n = 45)	154 ± 6 (n = 29)	
IZS, cryst.	B	U 40, 80				107 ± 15 b = 3.1[c] (n = 7)	
			0.27 ± 0.04 (n = 19)	2.0 ± 0.1 (n = 18)	6.8 ± 0.9 b = 0.2 (n = 43)	↑ P < 0.05 ↓	366 ± 18 (n = 9)
	P	U 40, 80			↑ P < 0.001 ↓	52 ± 19 b = 8.5 (n = 21) P < 0.01	
	H	U 40, 100		No data	11.3 ± 4.1 b = 0.2 (n = 8)	141 ± 38 b = 8.1 (n = 6)	
IZS, mix.	B/P, P, H	U 40, 80, 100	0.66 ± 0.08 (n = 74)				
	H	U 40, 100		2.2 ± 0.1 (n = 8) P < 0.02	10.3 ± 0.9 b = 0.17 (n = 23) P < 0.001	134 ± 24 b = 3.7 (n = 15) P < 0.001	517 ± 87 b = 12 (n = 11) P < 0.002
	P	U 40, 80, 100		1.5 ± 0.3 (n = 5)	6.2 ± 2.1 b = 0.15 (n = 7) P < 0.001	88 ± 12 b = 2.0 (n = 9)	365 ± 92 b = 15 (n = 15) n.s.
	B/P	U 40, 80, 100			12.7 ± 1.5 b = 0.13 (n = 10)		449 ± 15 (n = 8)

[a] Figures are the apparent rate constants ($\times 10^4$ month^{-1}) ± SE.
[b] B, bovine; P, porcine; H, human; B/P, mixture of bovine crystals and porcine amorphous phase.
[c] b values ($\times 10^4$), the coefficient to the quadratic term, are given when the polynomial expression gives the best fit of the time course.

(4) The rate of formation of HMWT products varies with the composition and formulation of the preparations and, in some cases, with the strength and species of insulin. Differences with respect to HMWT product formation can be observed within the same type of preparation from various manufacturers.

CID Formation

Covalent dimers are the main products formed in all preparations except for the protamine-containing preparations (NPH and PZI). In the neutral solutions the insulin molecules are associated mainly into noncovalent, Zn^{2+}-containing hexamers (5,11). The observation that the rate of formation of CID in the neutral solutions is independent of the insulin concentration strongly indicates that the intermolecular chemical reaction occurs mainly within the hexameric units, and not to any significant extent between the hexamers in the solution. As the crystalline and amorphous suspensions share with the solutions the hexamer as the common unit, CID is again most likely to arise mainly from intermolecular reactions within the hexamer in these preparations. This theory is supported by the fact that CID formation is of the same order of magnitude in neutral solution and in suspensions when these suspensions contain similar auxiliary substances (regular N1 versus IZS types).

It is normally assumed that chemical decomposition of drug suspensions takes place solely in the part of the drug in solution (12). In the IZS types of formulations the amount of insulin in solution is extremely small (<0.1 IU/ml) but the CID formation, nevertheless, occurs to the same extent as in the neutral solutions containing 100 IU/ml, indicating that the transformation reactions in these suspensions occur mainly within the solid crystalline phase. This is conceivable because the molecules in an insulin crystal have some conformational flexibility of their side chains and backbone for movements within the crystal lattice (13).

CID formation is generally fastest in preparations containing glycerol and phenol/cresol (regular N2 and NPH). Glycerol is well recognized to be able to stabilize proteins

Table III. Total HMWT Product Formation in Insulin Preparations Containing Dissolved Insulin[a]

Preparation	Species[b]	Strength	Temperature (°C)				
			4	15	25	37	45
Regular A2	P, B	U 40	9.3 ± 1.1 (n = 4)		102 ± 3 (n = 3)		
Regular N1	B	U 40, 80			15 ± 1 (n = 4) P < 0.001	104 ± 11 b = 1.7[c] (n = 7) P < 0.001	
	P, H	U 40–200	0.65 ± 0.06 (n = 33)	1.95 ± 0.13 (n = 39)	8.1 ± 0.2 (n = 67)	54 ± 6 b = 3.6 (n = 32)	186 ± 14 b = 4.5 (n = 33)
			N1 vs N2 (P, H) at all temperatures: P < 0.01				
Regular N2	P, H	U 40–500	1.64 ± 0.13 (n = 37)	3.5 ± 0.3 (n = 17)	11.2 ± 0.4 (n = 32)	140 ± 17 b = −12 (n = 25)	456 ± 56 b = −53 (n = 16)
Biphasic	P/B	U 40	0.95 ± 0.13 (n = 17)	3.5 ± 0.2 (n = 14)	11.9 ± 3.1 b = 0.36 (n = 23)	106 ± 20 b = 4.6 (n = 5)	

[a] Figures are the apparent first-order rate constants ($\times 10^4$ month^{-1}) ± SE.
[b] B, bovine; P, porcine; H, human; P/B, mixture of porcine dissolved and bovine crystalline insulin.
[c] b values ($\times 10^4$), the coefficient to the quadratic term, are given when the polynomial expression gives the best fit of the time course.

physically (14,15) and phenol has been demonstrated to enhance the stability of the insulin hexamer (16). It might be expected that such increased structural stability would result in diminished conformational flexibility and, consequently, decreased chemical reactivity as actually seen in the hydrolytic decomposition of insulin in the presence of phenol (1). However, glycerol at a high concentration has been shown to cause substantially increased formation of covalent insulin di- and polymers (17). Glycerolaldehyde, a potential impurity in glycerol formed by oxidation of the glycerol during

Table IV. Formation of Insulin Covalent Dimer and Covalent Insulin Protamine (CIP) Products in NPH Preparations[a]

Species[b]	Strength	Product	Temperature (°C)				
			4	15	25	37	45
P, H	U 40	Dimer	1.86 ± 0.17	8.3 ± 0.7	20.8 ± 0.8	127 ± 8 b = −12[c]	353 ± 24 b = −88
		CIP	2.54 ± 0.13	9.0 ± 0.6	23.5 ± 0.9	144 ± 10 b = −7	420 ± 51 b = −90
			(n = 27)	(n = 18)	(n = 38)	(n = 31)	(n = 6)
P	U 80	Dimer	1.60 ± 0.38	6.9 ± 0.4	12.9 ± 1.4		
		CIP	1.73 ± 0.31	6.8 ± 0.6	13.7 ± 1.6		
			(n = 9)	(n = 6)	(n = 9)		
P + H, U 40 vs U 100 (dimer and CIP):			n.s.		⊢−−−−−−−−−−−−−− P < 0.001 −−−−−−−−−−−−−−⊣		
P, H	U 100	Dimer	1.53 ± 0.22	4.3 ± 0.5	14.3 ± 1.0	69 ± 3	205 ± 23 b = −35
		CIP	2.4 ± 0.3	5.5 ± 0.5	18.1 ± 1.4	90 ± 3	257 ± 11 b = −56
			(n = 21)	(n = 15)	(n = 29)	(n = 20)	(n = 9)
P + H vs B (U 100)		CIP: n.s. at all temperatures					
		Dimer:	n.s.	P < 0.02	P < 0.001	P < 0.005	
B	U 100	Dimer	1.2 ± 0.3	2.5 ± 0.3	7.4 ± 0.8	41 ± 11	
		CIP	2.0 ± 0.4	4.9 ± 0.7	14 ± 1	75 ± 21	
			(n = 7)	(n = 7)	(n = 14)	(n = 5)	

[a] Figures are the apparent first-order rate constants ($\times 10^4$ month^{-1}) ± SE.
[b] P, porcine; H, human; B, bovine.
[c] b values ($\times 10^4$), the coefficient to the quadratic term, are given when the polynomial expression gives the best fit of the time course.

Table V. Formation of Insulin Covalent Dimer and Covalent Polymerization Products in Insulin Preparations[a]

Preparation	Species[b]	Product	Temperature (°C)		
			25	37	45
Regular N1	P, H	Dimers	6.4 ± 0.2	54 ± 3	177 ± 12
		Polymers	0.22 ± 0.02	1.7 ± 2	69 ± 6
			(n = 67)	(n = 32)	(n = 33)
IZS, amorph.	P, H	Dimers	5.0 ± 0.3	55 ± 2	97 ± 11
		Polymers	3.2 ± 0.3	92 ± 11	220 ± 16
			(n = 5)	(n = 13)	(n = 4)
IZS, cryst.	B, P	Dimers	8.0 ± 0.8	116 ± 4	
		Trimers	1.1 ± 0.2	29 ± 3	
		Tetramers		8 ± 2	
			(n = 43)	(n = 28)	

[a] Figures are the apparent rate constants ($\times 10^4$ month^{-1}) ± SE.
[b] B, bovine; P, porcine; H, human.

storage, is able to react chemically with amino groups through its carbonyl group under formation of Schiff base adducts. These reaction products are able to undergo Amadori rearrangement (18), which produces a new carbonyl function capable of forming Schiff base linkages with another amino group. Such reactions and subsequent rearrangement can therefore result in covalent cross-linking of proteins (18,19). Thus, in addition to the potential of forming CID by transamidation reactions (10), the CID can also be generated via an initial reaction with glycerol degradation products. The decrease in CID (and CIP product) formation with increasing insulin strength in the NPH preparation clearly indicates involvement of the auxiliary substances, as the concentration of excipient relative to that of insulin decreases with increasing strength of the preparation.

The rate of CID formation seems to increase with time in the preparations containing methylparaben (positive b values), whereas a more constant or declining rate with time applies to the preparations with phenol as preservative. As CID formation at neutral reactions increases with falling pH (unpublished observation), this difference is consistent with the fact that pH changes to lower values during storage of the preparations containing methylparaben as preservative agent (5).

CIP Formation

Although the content of protamine in the NPH crystals corresponds to only 0.15 protamine molecule per insulin monomer, the chemical reaction between protamine and insulin proceeds in the NPH preparation at a rate slightly higher than the rate of CID formation (Table IV). Protamine from salmon (salmine), used in the preparations, does not contain asparaginyl or glutaminyl residues, nor does it include side-chain amine groups (Lys) in the sequence. It is therefore able to participate in transamidation or Schiff base-mediated reactions only with its N-terminal amino group, but because protamine has great conformational flexibility within the crystal lattice (Dodson, personal communication), its N terminal has the capacity to react with insulin by intermolecular aminolysis, resulting in transamidation between the molecules.

Table VI. Effect of Concentration on Formation of HMWT Products in Regular N1[a]

Concentration	Temperature (°C)					
	25		37		45	
	Dimers	Oligo- & polymers	Dimers	Oligo- & polymers	Dimers	Oligo- & polymers
U 40	6.6	0.2	52	0.6	139	23
		(n = 53)		(n = 26)		(n = 16)
U 80	6.3	1.4	48	3.9		
		(n = 8)		(n = 3)		
U 100	1.5	1.3	73	18	171	69
		(n = 4)		(n = 3)		(n = 10)
U 500					214	78
						(n = 7)
Conc. effect	n.s.	P < 0.05	n.s.	n.s.	n.s.	n.s.

[a] Figures are the apparent rate constants ($\times 10^4$ month^{-1}).

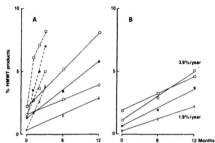

Fig. 4. Formation of HMWT products in human insulin preparations from four manufacturers during storage at 25°C (——) or 37°C (– – – –). Manufacturer 1 (●); 2 (□); 3 (○); 4 (×). (A) NPH insulin: 40 IU/ml (● and □); 100 IU/ml (× and ○). (B) Regular N2: all 100 IU/ml.

Covalent Oligo- and Polymer Formation

The covalent trimers and tetramers formed in IZS preparations are most likely products of continued transamidation. In comparison, the formation of covalent polymer in the neutral solutions and in the preparations with amorphously precipitated insulin (IZS, amorph.) seems to occur in parallel with the formation of CID, probably as a result of disulfide interchange (10). Such reactions are catalyzed by thiols, which can arise by initial hydrolytic cleavage of disulfides or via beta-elimination in neutral and alkaline media (20). Intermolecular disulfide exchange requires closeness between disulfide bridges from different insulin molecules. This is not the case within the hexamer or when hexamers pack in the rhombohedral (IZS cryst. preparations) or monoclinic (NPH) crystals. It is therefore not surprising that covalent polymerization due to disulfide reshuffling is undetectable in these types of preparations. However, such reaction becomes possible when the individual hexamers are capable of approaching one another in a random way as in solution or when the insulin is amorphously precipitated. The increasing oligo- and polymer formation with increasing insulin concentration in regular N solutions (Fig. 2 and Table VI) indicates that the reaction takes place between different hexamers in the neutral solution.

Whereas the initial disulfide lysis is a slow process, and therefore rate determining, the subsequent interchange reactions are fast, and as every single interchange leaves a new highly reactive thiolate ion, the initial hydrolysis starts a chain reaction resulting in accelerating polymer formation. Thus, the accumulation of CID and covalent oligomers as a result of disulfide interchange is expected to be low, as also revealed by the low proportion of these products after storage at temperatures at which these processes prevail.

Influence of HMWT Products on the Quality of Preparations

The formation of HMWT products in commercial insulin preparations is generally much slower than the chemical decomposition of the insulin as a result of hydrolytic reactions taking place during storage (1). The impact on the quality and therapeutic usefulness of the preparations might, however, be more serious. Thus, some of the immunological side effects associated with insulin therapy may be due to the presence of covalent aggregates of insulin in the therapeutical preparations (21–23), and specific antibodies against CID have been identified in 30% of insulin-treated diabetic patients (21). Recently cutaneous allergic manifestations resulting from the cell-mediated hypersensitivity response to CID have been reported and the response to stimulation of allergic patients' lymphocytes by commercial insulin preparations was demonstrated to vary with the content of CID in the preparations. A CID level of 2% generated a highly significant response, whereas no significant response was seen when the CID content was between 0.3 and 0.6% (23). Therefore, in order to minimize the frequency of clinical allergic reactions, the content of CID should be kept as low as possible, preferably below 1%. Times to formation of 1% of HMWT products during storage of some of the preparations are shown in Table VII.

The significance of the CIP product in relation to immunological side effects of insulin treatment is unresolved. More than one-third of diabetic subjects treated with NPH have circulating antibodies against protamine (24), and the presence of such antibodies as well as of insulin antibodies might be connected with the content of the CIP products in NPH.

Table VII. Times to Formation of 1% of HMWT Products in Different Preparations (Months)[a]

Preparation	Species	Temperature (°C)			
		4	15	25	37
Regular N1	Human, porcine	154	51	12	1.7
Regular N2	Human, porcine	61	29	9	1.3
NPH (U 100)	Human, porcine	25	10	3.6	0.6
IZS, amorphous	Porcine	357	83	13	0.6
IZS, crystalline	Bovine	370	50	11	0.9
	Human	370	No data	5.2	No data
IZS, mixed	Human	152	45	8.5	0.7

[a] The figures are calculated using the rate data from Tables I–III.

ACKNOWLEDGMENTS

The authors wish to acknowledge the skillful technical assistance of Lene Grønlund Andersen, Lene Bramsen, Lise Frank, Jessie Frederiksen, Lone Jørgensen, Anne-Marie Kolstrup, Eva Bøg Kristensen, Harriet Markussen, Birgit Dræby Spon, and Dorthe Stütz. We are grateful to Klaus Jørgensen, Novo Research Institute, and Professor Francis C. Szoka, Jr., University of California, San Francisco, for critically reading the manuscript and for helpful comments. We also thank Kathleen Larsen for help with preparing the manuscript.

REFERENCES

1. J. Brange, L. Langkjær, S. Havelund, and A. Vølund. Chemical stability of insulin. 1. Hydrolytic degradation during storage of pharmaceutical preparations. *Pharm Res.* 9:715–726 (1992).
2. J. Schlichtkrull, M. Pingel, L. G. Heding, J. Brange, and K. H. Jørgensen. Insulin preparations with prolonged effect. In A. Hasselblatt and F. von Bruchhausen (eds.), *Handbook of Experimental Pharmacology, New Series, Vol. XXXII/2*, Springer-Verlag, Berlin, Heidelberg, New York, 1975, pp. 729–777.
3. J. Brange, L. Langkjær, S. Havelund, and E. Sørensen. Chemical stability of insulin: Neutral insulin solutions. *Diabetologia* 25:193 (1983) (abstr).
4. J. Brange, L. Langkjær, S. Havelund, and E. Sørensen. Chemical stability of insulin: Formation of covalent insulin dimers and other higher molecular weight transformation products in intermediate- and long-acting insulin preparations. *Diabetologia* 27:259A–260A (1984) (abstr).
5. J. Brange, B. Skelbaek-Pedersen, L. Langkjaer, U. Damgaard, H. Ege, S. Havelund, L. G. Heding, K. H. Jørgensen, J. Lykkeberg, J. Markussen, M. Pingel, and E. Rasmussen. *Galenics of Insulin: The Physico-chemical and Pharmaceutical Aspects of Insulin and Insulin Preparations*, Springer-Verlag, Berlin, Heidelberg, New York, London, Paris, Tokyo, 1987.
6. D. F. Steiner, O. Hallund, A. Rubenstein, S. Cho, and C. Bayliss. Isolation and properties of proinsulin, intermediate forms, and other minor components from crystalline bovine insulin. *Diabetes* 17:725–736 (1968).
7. D. F. Steiner. Proinsulin and the biosynthesis of insulin. *N. Engl. J. Med.* 280:1106–1113 (1969).
8. H.-J. Helbig. *Insulindimere aus der b-Komponente von Insulinpräparationen*, Dissertation, Rheinish-Westfälische Technische Hochschule, Aachen, 1976.
9. T. R. Csorba, H. G. Gattner, and P. Cuatrecasas. Partial dimerization of insulin. *Clin. Res.* 20:918 (1972) (abstr).
10. J. Brange. Insulin transformation products formed during storage of insulin preparations: Isolation, characterization and properties (in preparation).
11. J. Brange, D. R. Owens, S. Kang, and A. Vølund. Monomeric insulins and their experimental and clinical implications. *Diabetes Care* 13:923–954 (1990).
12. J. T. Carstensen. *Drug Stability: Principles and Practices*, Dekker, New York and Basel, 1990.
13. E. N. Baker, T. L. Blundell, J. F. Cutfield, S. M. Cutfield, E. J. Dodson, G. G. Dodson, D. M. C. Hodgkin, R. E. Hubbard, N. W. Isaacs, C. D. Reynolds, K. Sakabe, N. Sakabe, and N. M. Vijayan. The structure of 2Zn pig insulin crystals at 1.5 Å resolution. *Phil. Trans. R. Soc.* 319:369–456 (1988).
14. J. F. Back, D. Oakenfull, and M. B. Smith. Increased thermal stability of proteins in the presence of sugars and polyols. *Biochemistry* 18:5191–5196 (1979).
15. K. Gekko and S. N. Timasheff. Mechanism of protein stabilization by glycerol: Preferential hydration in glycerol-water mixtures. *Biochemistry* 20:4667–4676 (1981).
16. U. Derewenda, Z. Derewenda, E. J. Dodson, G. G. Dodson, C. D. Reynolds, G. D. Smith, C. Sparks, and D. Swenson. Phenol stabilizes more helix in a new symmetrical zinc insulin hexamer. *Nature* 338:594–596 (1989).
17. J. Brange, S. Havelund, P. Hansen, L. Langkjær, E. Sørensen, and P. Hildebrandt. Formulation of physically stable neutral solutions for continuous infusion by delivery systems. In J. L. Gueriguian, E. D. Bransome, and A. S. Outschoorn (eds.), *Hormone Drugs*, US Pharmacopoeial Convention, Rockville, MD, 1982, pp. 96–105.
18. A. S. Acharya and J. M. Manning. Reaction of glycolaldehyde with proteins: Latent crosslinking potential of α-hydroxyaldehydes. *Proc. Natl. Acad. Sci. USA* 80:3590–3594 (1983).
19. J. Bello and H. R. Bello. Chemical modification and crosslinking of proteins by impurities in glycerol. *Arch. Biochem. Biophys.* 172:608–610 (1976).
20. M. C. Manning, K. Patel, and R. T. Borchardt. Stability of protein pharmaceuticals. *Pharm. Res.* 6:903–918 (1989).
21. D. C. Robbins, S. M. Cooper, S. E. Fineberg, and P. M. Mead. Antibodies to covalent aggregates of insulin in blood of insulin-using diabetic patients. *Diabetes* 36:838–841 (1987).
22. M. Maislos, P. M. Mead, D. H. Gaynor, and D. C. Robbins. The source of the circulating aggregate of insulin in type I diabetic patients is therapeutic insulin. *J. Clin. Invest.* 77:717–723 (1986).
23. R. E. Ratner, T. M. Phillips, and M. Steiner. Persistent cutaneous insulin allergy resulting from high-molecular-weight insulin aggregates. *Diabetes* 39:728–733 (1990).
24. L. J. Nell and J. W. Thomas. Frequency and specificity of protamine antibodies in diabetic and control subjects. *Diabetes* 37:172–176 (1988).

Reproduced from *Acta Pharmaceutica Nordica*, 4(4):149–158,
1992. Copyright Swedish Pharmaceutical Society. With permission.

Chemical stability of insulin

3. Influence of excipients, formulation, and pH

J. Brange* and L. Langkjær

Novo Research Institute, Novo Alle, DK-2880 Bagsværd, Denmark

The influence of auxiliary substances and pH on the chemical transformations of insulin in pharmaceutical
formulation, including various hydrolytic and intermolecular cross-linking reactions, was studied. Bacteriostatic agents had a profound stabilizing effect – phenol > *m*-cresol > methylparaben – on deamidation as
well as on insulin intermolecular cross-linking reactions. Of the isotonicity substances, NaCl generally had
a stabilizing effect whereas glycerol and glucose led to increased chemical deterioration. Phenol and sodium chloride exerted their stabilizing effect through independent mechanisms. Zinc ions, in concentrations that promote association of insulin into hexamers, increase the stability, whereas higher zinc content
had no further influence. Protamine gave rise to additional formation of covalent protamine-insulin products which increased with increasing protamine concentration. The impact of excipients on the chemical
processes seems to be dictated mainly via an influence on the three-dimensional insulin structure. The effect
of the physical state of the insulin on the chemical stability was also complex, suggesting an intricate dependence of intermolecular proximity of involved functional groups. At pH values below five and above eight,
insulin degrades relatively fast. At acid pH, deamidation at residue A21 and covalent insulin dimerization
dominates, whereas disulfide reactions leading to covalent polymerization and formation of A- and B-
chains prevailed in alkaline medium. Structure-reactivity relationship is proposed to be a main determinant
for the chemical transformation of insulin.

Insulin is one of the most extensively studied biomolecules and has been the subject of pioneering work on
protein primary and three-dimensional structure, as
well as chemical synthesis. Notwithstanding its medical
importance and the availability of a large number of different pharmaceutical preparations, only sparse information is available on the chemical stability of insulin in
such formulations. In two previous articles in this series,
the quantitative aspects of the chemical stability of insulin in pharmaceutical formulation have been reported in
terms of hydrolytic degradation [1] and insulin intermolecular transformation reactions leading to higher molecular weight products [2].

Whereas hydrolytic degradation in acid medium is
due to deamidation at Asn^{A21} [3], it was found that the
deamidation around neutral reaction takes place at residue B3 with formation of a mixture of isoAsp and Asp
derivatives [4, 1]. This transformation of insulin into two
different B3 derivatives involves the formation of a
cyclic imide intermediate which hydrolyzes either under
retention of a normal peptide linkage corresponding to
simple deamidation or of a beta-carboxyl linkage (isopeptide). The rate of hydrolysis at B3 varies with the
composition and the physical state of the insulin in the
formulation.

In certain crystalline suspensions, an insulin species-
dependent cleavage of the peptide bond A8–A9 was
observed. The hydrolytic cleavage of the peptide backbone takes place only in preparations containing rhombohedral zinc insulin crystals in addition to free zinc ions
[1].

The higher molecular weight transformation
(HMWT) products formed during storage were mainly
covalent insulin dimers (CID), but in protamine-containing preparations a concurrent formation of covalent
insulin-protamine products (CIPP) takes place. During
storage at ≥ 25°C parallel or consecutive formation of
covalent oligo- and polymers can also be observed in
certain preparations. The rate of HMWT is only slightly influenced by the species of insulin but varies with
composition and formulation. CIDs are formed between molecules in the insulin dimeric or hexameric
units common for all types of preparations, mainly
through transamidation reactions (aminolysis) by the B-
chain N-terminal amine group on Asn side chains of the
A-chain [2, 5–7].

In the present paper the influence of pH and of the
different excipients on the chemical transformation is
studied in greater detail. Kinetics and mechanisms of

---

* Correspondence

95

the various insulin transformation reactions will be discussed more specifically in a following communication.

Experimental

Materials

The insulins used for the studies were monocomponent (MC) insulin of different species (porcine, bovine and human). Potency: 28 IU/mg (dry weight) corresponding to 1.68×10^8 IU/mol. Zn^{2+} content (unless otherwise stated): 0.4% (w/w of insulin) corresponding to approximately 2 Zn^{2+} per insulin hexamer. Zinc-free insulins contained < 0.01% Zn^{2+} (< 0.01 mol per mol insulin). Insulin: purity > 99% by reversed-phase HPLC. The content of impurities was: Desamidoinsulins: nondetectable (< 0.2%) by disc electrophoresis [1]. Di- and polymerization products: < 0.2% as detected by size exclusion chromatography [2].

Distilled water was used for the preparation of electrophoretic buffers and chromatographic eluents. All other chemicals used were either official (Ph. Eur. or B. P.) or analytical grade. The percentages are given as w/v, except for degradation products which are w/w of the initial insulin content.

Handling and analytical procedures

Preparation, storage and isolation of samples for analytical measurements were performed as described earlier [1]. Adjustment to final pH was made with special care to avoid local, larger pH fluctuations, resulting in unwanted insulin phase changes. Readings of pH were carried out on a Radiometer instrument (Type PHM 64) at 20°C using combined glass electrodes. Quantitative estimation of the content of hydrolysis products was performed by disc electrophoresis and densitometric scanning or by reversed-phase HPLC (RP-HPLC) as described earlier [1]. The content of degradation (lower molecular transformation) products or of higher molecular transformation (HMWT) products was estimated by either conventional size exclusion chromatography (CSEC) or by high performance size exclusion chromatography (HPSEC), as described earlier [2]. Statistical analyses were performed as described earlier [2].

Results and discussion

The excipients used in pharmaceutical preparations of insulin can be classified into bacteriostatic agents (phenol, m-cresol or methylparaben), isotonicity substances (glucose, glycerol or sodium chloride), buffering substances (phosphate, TRIS or acetate), and excipients used to provide a sustained release of insulin from the product (protamine sulfate, Zn^{2+} or both). A gradation of protracted effect is also obtained by varying the physical state of the insulin, i.e. soluble, amorphous or different types of insulin crystals. As the type of degradation products formed, and the rate of decomposition was found to vary not only with the composition and formulation of the pharmaceutical preparations but also

with the physical state, including the crystal type of the insulin [1, 2] it was of interest to study the specific influence of such factors on the chemical stability.

Effect of excipients

In order to explore the particular effect of the various excipients on the chemical stability, the type and concentration of preservative, isotonicity and buffering substances were individually varied in a series of experiments. The results of accelerated degradation studies are presented in Tables 1–3 and Fig. 1. The type of isotonic agent and of preservative has a profound effect on the extent of deamidation as well as the formation of HMWT products. There is a clear gradation in the stabilizing effect of the preservatives: Phenol > m-cresol > methylparaben, and of the isotonic agents: NaCl > glycerol > glucose (Tables 1 and 2). Phenol and NaCl apparently exert their stabilizing influence through an independent mechanism since an additive effect of the two compounds is observed when they are used together, with phenol having the individually largest effect (Table 3, Fig. 1). The optimal effect is obtained at or below the actual concentrations used in the present official preparations (Fig. 1), so the use of e.g. a higher phenol concentration for improving the chemical stability would not be of any benefit. None of the present commercial preparations actually utilizes the combination of sodium

Table 1. *Influence of different combinations of excipients on the chemical transformation of insulin in neutral solution.*
A. *Deamidation*

	glycerol (1.6%)	NaCl (0.7%)
phenol (0.2%)	21.1 (± 1.2)	6.1 (± 0.4)
m-cresol (0.3%)	28.1 (± 4.0)	10.0 (± 0.8)
methylparaben (0.1%)		32.1 (± 2.7)

The figures are the mean percentage (SEM, n=3–6) formed of total monodesamido-(B3)-insulin after storage for 2 years at 25°C.

B. *Covalent dimerization*

	glycerol (1.6%)	NaCl (0.7%)
phenol (0.2%)	4.3	0.30
m-cresol (0.3%)	5.0	0.69
methylparaben (0.1%)		0.74

The figures are single estimates of the amount formed (%) of CID after storage of the solutions (40 IU/ml) for 2 months at 37°C.

C. *Formation of covalent HMWT products*

	CID	oligo- & polymer	total HMWT
phenol (0.2%)	2.4	0.5	2.9
methylparaben (0.1%)	4.0	2.1	6.1

The figures are single estimates of the amount formed (%) after storage for 3 months at 37°C of preparations (100 IU/ml) containing glycerol as isotonicity substance.

chloride and phenol, and an experimental neutral insulin solution containing 0.2% phenol and 0.7% NaCl was therefore tested. The results obtained (Table 4) con-

Table 2. *Influence of buffering substances and other additives on the deamidation of insulin in neutral solution.*
A. *Buffer and preservatives*

Preservative	Buffering substance		
	acetate (10 mM)	phosphate (13 mM)	none
none	47.0 (2.0)		
methylparaben (0.1%)	24.2 (1.9)		
m-cresol (0.3%)	11.3 (0.6)	9.3 (0.5)	10.5 (0.6)
phenol (0.2%)	6.0 (0.3)	7.0 (0.4)	6.2 (0.4)

The figures are the total deamidation (%) at residue B3 (isoAsp and Asp derivatives) during storage for 2 years at 25°C of neutral solutions (pH 7.4) which also contained 0.7% NaCl. The ratio of isoAsp/Asp derivatives are shown in parentheses.

B. *Buffer and isotonicity substances*

Isotonicity substance	Buffering substance	
	10 mM acetate	40 mM TRIS
NaCl (0.7%)	14.1%	12.6%
glycerol (1.6%)	28.4%	
glucose (5%)	51.5%	

The figures are the total deamidation (%) at residue B3 during storage for 6 months at 25°C of neutral solutions (pH 7.4) which also contained 0.1% methylparaben.

Table 3. *Individual stabilizing effects of phenol and NaCl on the deamidation of insulin in neutral solution.*

Sodium chloride concentration (%)	Phenol concentration (%)	
	0	0.2
0	23.5	10.0
0.7	15.4	1.5

The figures are the total deamidation (%) at B3 (isoAsp and Asp derivatives) during storage for 2 months at 37°C.

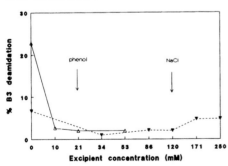

Fig. 1. *The influence of excipient concentration on deamidation of insulin in neutral regular solution.*
Phenol ($\triangle$—$\triangle$) and sodium chloride ($\blacktriangledown$ - - - $\blacktriangledown$) concentrations were varied in solutions of porcine insulin (40 IU/ml, pH 7.4) containing the normal concentrations of sodium chloride (0.7% ~ 120 mM) and phenol (0.2% ~ 21 mM), respectively. These concentrations are indicated with arrows in the figure storage for 1 year at 25°C.

Table 4. *Influence of composition on the chemical transformation of insulin in neutral solution.*

Formulation	CID formation				B3 deamidation	
	4°C	15°C	25°C	37°C	4°C	25°C
Regular I	0.65	2.0	8.1	54	18	210
	± 0.06	± 0.1	± 0.2	± 6	± 2	± 20
Regular II					11	114
					± 2	± 15
Regular experimental	1.2	3.8	9.5	37	N.D.	23
	± 0.2	± 0.4	± 0.7	± 4		± 4

The figures represent the observed first-order rate constants ($\times 10^4$ month^{-1}) ± SE. N. D.= not detectable.
Regular I and II data are from Refs. 1 and 2.
All formulations contained porcine insulin (40 IU/ml). Regular I was formulated with methylparaben (0.1%) and NaCl (0.7%), II with phenol (0.2%) and glycerol (1.6%), and the experimental formulation with phenol (0.2%) and NaCl (0.7%).

firmed a substantially increased resistance with respect to deamidation of this formulation, as compared to the two commercial preparations. The rate of CID formation was also reduced during storage at 37°C, as observed earlier with this combination (Table 1B), but at the lower temperatures significantly increased formation of CID occurs compared to the official preparation. This observation seriously questions the relevancy of using accelerated degradation studies in predicting protein stability at lower temperatures.

Preservative effect

The profound stabilizing effect of the different preservatives (Tables 1 and 2 A) is presumably related to the recently discovered insulin structural changes promoted by phenol and its derivatives [8, 9]. This structural transformation involves formation of an additional helical segment in the B-chain N-terminal within which the deamidation takes place. In addition, the phenol molecules sit in cavities between dimers in the hexamer and make van der Waal's contact with His[B5], which increases the structural stability in this region [9]. The ranking of the stabilizing effect of phenol, and its derivatives correlates with the CD-spectral changes seen in the far ultraviolet region [8]. This strongly indicates that the degree of stabilization is associated with the extent of structural change in the B-chain N-terminal. A concomitant reduction in the B3 isoAsp/Asp ratio implies either increased direct deamidation of the side chain amide group or change in local structure around the hydrolyzing intermediate imide when the structure is stabilized by phenol or phenol derivatives. Such conformational difference could result in reduced accessibility to hydrolysis of the succinimide peptide linkage of the imide (isoAsp formation) because of steric hindrance, or increased susceptibility of the imide β-peptide linkage to hydrolysis (Asp formation) due to a catalytic effect by juxtaposed functional groups in the three-dimensional structure [10].

Formation of HMWT products is also reduced when phenol rather than *m*-cresol or, especially, methylparaben is used as preservative (Table 1 B and C). This effect probably reflects the fact that the primarily reacting B-chain N-terminal [10] becomes buried within the insulin hexamer by the phenol-promoted switch into an α-helix [9].

Recently, the binding of phenolic ligands to hexameric insulin was studied using microcalorimetry and NMR spectroscopy [11, 12]. A combination of van der Waal's interactions, hydrophobic effects, and protein conformational changes appeared to be involved in the binding of such ligands. One binding site per insulin monomer was observed and it is therefore uncertain whether other binding sites in the hexamer apart from those mentioned above, were involved. However, in this respect it is interesting to note that in acid solution, with no hexamer to encompass the ligand, there might also be a stabilizing effect of phenol with respect to the formation of the A21 monodesamido product [1].

Influence of isotonicity substance

It has been demonstrated for model peptides [13–15] as well as for proteins [16] that deamidation proceeds faster with increasing ionic strength. The same tendency is observed for neutral insulin solutions in the range 0.2–1.5% (0.03–0.3 M) NaCl, whereas a decrease in deamidation is seen when the NaCl concentration is changed from < 0.05–0.2% (< 0.01 to 0.03 M) (Fig. 1). In this context, it should be mentioned that in other studies no effect of ionic strength could be found [17, 18]. It is conceivable that the effect of ionic strength is mediated by an influence of electrostatic interactions on the local conformation around the deamidating residue. Such an impact may make the intramolecular imide formation (rate limiting step) at B3 conformationally more or less favorable [10].

The use of glycerol as excipient clearly has a deteriorating effect on the chemical stability of insulin in neutral formulation, not only with respect to deamidation (Table 2 B) but also due to increased formation of covalent di- and polymers (Table 1 B and C; refs. 2, 19). This latter effect is probably caused primarily by aldehyde impurities in the glycerol [20]. These react with insulin amino groups under the formation of Schiff bases, with a subsequent Amadori rearrangement followed by new similar reactions [21]. The end result is covalent cross-linking of the insulin [2, 10]. The combination of glycerol with methylparaben clearly exhibits the most deteriorating effect (Table 1 C). This can reasonably be ascribed to the relatively greater mobility of the B-chain N-terminal in the presence of methylparaben, as compared to phenol and *m*-cresol, increasing its potential for Schiff base formation. Glucose, used as isotonic agent in acid insulin solutions, has the same capacity at neutral to alkaline reaction to react via its aldehyde function with formation of Schiff base and has, accordingly, also been shown to increase the formation of HMWT products in neutral insulin solutions [22]. Interestingly, also B3 deamidation is substantially increased in the presence of glycerol or glucose. This effect may be attributed to the above-mentioned influence of minimal ion strength and, in addition, the tendency of polyhydric alcohols in low concentration to loosen the globular structure of proteins [23]. The effect was found to correlate with the number of hydroxymethyl groups per molecule of solute, which is consistent with the observed greater effect of glucose as compared to glycerol (Table 2 B). This may, however, also be related to the higher molar concentration of glucose. The denaturating effects may render the B-chain N-terminal more flexible and facilitate the intermediate B3 imide formation.

Stability results obtained with two different neutral soluble formulations [1] are in keeping with the observed effects of the individual excipients. Since the deterioration due to glycerol in Regular II (with phenol or cresol) is more than counterbalanced by the stabilizing effect due to phenol or *m*-cresol, the formation of deamidation products in this preparation is less than that in Regular I (with methylparaben+NaCl).

Effect of buffer

Deamidation of oligo peptides [13, 14, 24] and of proteins [15, 18] has been reported to depend markedly on buffer type and concentration. Particularly the use of phosphate buffer under neutral or alkaline conditions was emphasized as enhancing the rate of deamidation five times more than e.g. tris buffer [13, 14]. However, others were not able to detect any buffer catalysis in deamidation of an Asn tetrapeptide by changing the phosphate concentration from 0 to 50 mM [25]. The three different buffering substances, in the concentrations used in current neutral insulin solutions, have very little influence, if any, on neutral deamidation of insulin (Table 2 A and B).

Effect of zinc ions

Two zinc ions per six insulin molecules are required for the assembly of insulin into a hexamer, which is the predominant structural unit in all neutral insulin preparations [7]. Although an increase of the normal 2 Zn^{2+} per hexamer of insulin in neutral solution to 4 Zn^{2+} per hexamer of insulin has been shown physically to have a stabilizing effect on the hexameric structure [26], it does not seem to change the chemical stability of the insulin. Apparently, the extra zinc ions strengthen the hexameric assembly without influencing the conformation flexibility of the B-chain N-terminal residues involved in both B3 deamidation and CID formation [10]. This is plausible because the additional zinc ions mainly act by neutralizing repulsive charges in the center of the hexamer [27]. In contrast, when insulin is formulated in neutral solution without any zinc content, and the main association state changes from 6 to about 3–4 insulin mole-

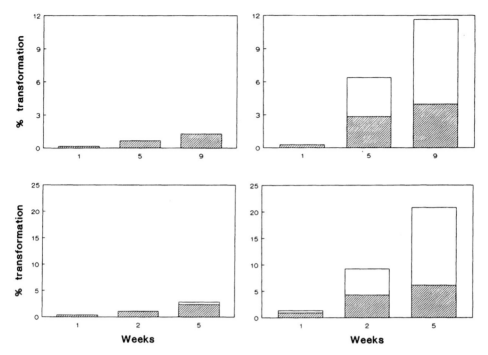

Fig. 2. Effect of zinc ions on the formation of covalent insulin dimers (hatched bars) and polymers (open bars) in neutral solutions (porcine insulin 40 IU/ml, methylparaben 0.1%, NaCl 0.7%, pH 7.4).
Left panels: insulin containing 2 Zn^{2+} per hexamer. Right panels: zinc-free insulin. Top panels: storage at 37°C. Bottom panels: storage at 45°C.

cules at normal pharmaceutical concentrations (40–100 IU/ml) [28], the tendency to formation of covalent HMWT products is substantially increased. As demonstrated in Fig. 2, the reduced stability of zinc-free insulin is, in particular, due to a dramatically elevated formation of covalent insulin polymers. Insulin polymer formation has been demonstrated to be primarily due to disulfide exchange reactions, which require closeness between disulfide bridges from different insulin molecules [10]. This is not the case within the 2 Zn^{2+} hexamer. It is therefore not surprising that covalent polymerization is absent or very low in the zinc ion-containing neutral solutions, as disulfide reshuffling would require reaction between different hexameric units in the solution. In contrast, in neutral insulin solutions devoid of zinc, the dimeric to tetrameric units [29] probably make random, close interactions which increase the possibility for disulfide interchange between dimeric units.

Effect of protamine

In all protamine-containing preparations an additional peak of HMWT product, eluting in front of the peak containing the CID products, can be observed when aged samples of the preparations are analyzed by size exclusion chromatography [2, 7]. Amino acid analysis has revealed that this peak contains a reaction product consisting of one insulin and one protamine molecule, probably linked through the N-terminal of protamine with the A-chain of insulin [30]. The amount formed of such covalent insulin protamine products (CIPP) in the isophane (NPH) type of preparation is normally slightly higher than that of the concurrently formed CID [2]. The rate of CIPP formation is substantially increased when the protamine content relative to insulin is increased as in the Protamine Zinc Insulin preparation [2]. The same tendency is observed in NPH when a slightly increased protamine/insulin ratio is required to obtain the isophane ratio [7] at higher pH values (see below).

Influence of formulation (insulin physical state)

As a consequence of the individual effects of the various excipients, the composition of the preparations has a significant but complex influence on the chemical stabi-

Table 5. *Influence of method of preparation of IZS amorphous on the chemical transformation of insulin.*

Preparation method	B3 deamidation		Formation of HMWT products		
	15°C	25°C	15°C	25°C	37°C
official	0.77	2.2	0.01	0.08	1.5
experimental	0.32	1.2	0.06	0.34	4.9

The figures are the observed first-order rate constants ($\times 10^2$ month^{-1}). The experimental preparation was prepared with a simple change in mixing order of the individual constituents (see text).

lity of insulin. Equally important is the physical state of insulin in the preparation since insulin in crystalline form tends to be more stable than insulin in amorphous or dissolved form [1, 2]. However, chemical stability is not a simple function of the rigidity and aggregation state of the insulin molecules. Proximity of potentially interacting groups is also important. Thus, the overall hydrolytic stability of bovine, crystalline Insulin Zinc Suspension (IZS, crystalline) at 25°C is actually worse than that of an insulin solution with an almost identical composition [1]. Deamidation in such crystalline suspensions is very slow but when the suspension contains rhombohedral zinc insulin crystals in addition to a high Zn^{2+} content, a hydrolytic cleavage of the A-chain between residue A8 and A9, catalytically assisted by residues from an adjacent hexamer, can be observed [1, 31]. The stability of insulin in amorphous suspension is generally similar to that of dissolved insulin but at storage temperatures > 25°C, covalent polymer formation is faster in amorphous insulin [2]. In unique cases, there seems to be an effect also of the method of preparation on the chemical stability. Thus, in an experimental IZS, amorphous preparation with the same final composition as the official preparation, but prepared with a single change in mixing order, the chemical stability changed drastically (Table 5). The rate of formation of B3 transformation products was only half of that observed in the official preparation. In contrast, the propensity for formation of HMWT products, mainly due to disulfide exchange [30], was significantly increased in the experimental preparation. The amorphous precipitate in the latter formulation was less voluminous, implying a closer packing of the hexamers in the amorphous precipitate. As the disulfide exchanges are inter-hexamer reactions [2], the closer approach between hexamers makes disulfide reactions more likely.

Chemical stability as a function of pH

Hydrolysis

We have previously reported that hydrolytic decomposition of insulin takes place at different sites in the molecule under acid and neutral conditions [1]. At acid pH, Asn^{A21}, the C-terminal residue of the A-chain, is particularly labile [3] and 20–30% deamidation of this residue occurs during storage of an acid (pH 3) preparation for one year at 4°C [7]. Around neutral pH, dea-

midation is much slower and takes place exclusively at residue Asn^{B3}, with an intermediate formation of a succinimide which hydrolyzes by two pathways to yield a mixture of α- and β-aspartyl-(B3)-insulin [1, 4, 30].

To acquire more detailed knowledge of the influence of pH on insulin chemical transformation, different insulin formulations were studied over a wide range of pH. As insulin is only slightly soluble around its isoelectric point (pI 5.4), suspensions of amorphous or crystalline insulin were also included in these investigations.

Hydrolysis of porcine insulin as a function of pH in the acid range is shown in Table 6. Progressive deamidation with formation of mono-, di-, tri- and tetradesamidoinsulins is observed with decreasing pH. However, significant amounts of didesamidoinsulin first appear after formation of 80% of monodesamidoinsulin, confirming the extreme lability of the Asn^{A21} amido group with respect to acid hydrolysis [3], even in more diluted acids. Deamidation at A21 is probably catalyzed by the uncharged C-terminal carboxylgroup [10, 32, 33], involving a proton transfer to the amide group followed by a nucleophilic attack by the carboxylate function [34]. Therefore, the rate of hydrolysis can be expected to be a function of the degree of protonation of the terminal α-carboxylgroup. Accordingly, the rate of deamidation of insulin increases with decreasing pH in the pH interval from 5 to 3 (Fig. 3). The further increase in the rate of total deamidation in the pH interval 3–1.5, in which the C-terminal carboxyl group is virtually fully protonated, can probably be ascribed to additional hydronium ion-catalyzed deamidation of all 6 amide groups in the molecule, as actually indicated by the data (Table 6). The observation that insulin deamidates at A21 at an appreciable rate even around pH 5 (Fig. 3), with relatively small fractions of the α-carboxyl groups protonated, can possibly be ascribed to the fact that the A21 carboxylate in the crystal structure is seen to form an intramolecular salt bridge to Arg^{B22} [35]. This might facilitate the catalytic proton transfer to the amide group even at relatively high pH. In this connection, it should be mentioned that deamidation proceeds in slightly acid crystalline suspension at essentially the

Table 6. *Deamidation as a function of pH in acid medium.*

Desamido-insulin (DI) derivative	pH			
	1.5	2.0	3.0	3.0 +Zn
Mono-DI	3.2	35.7	78.4	79.7
Di-DI	21.1	36.1	2.0	3.3
Tri-DI	32.9	20.8		
Tetra- DI	42.8	2.1		
Total deamidation	100	94.7	80.4	82.0

The figures are estimates by disc electrophoresis plus scanning [1] of the amounts formed (%) after storage of porcine insulin (40 IU/ml, methylparaben: 0.1%, NaCl: 0.7%, ±1 mM Zn^{2+}) at the respective pH values for 6 years at 4°C.

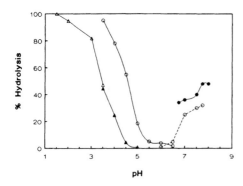

Fig. 3. *Influence of pH on the hydrolytic degradation of insulin.*

Acid solutions of bovine insulin (40 IU/ml, methylparaben 0.1%, NaCl 0.7%) were stored for 6 years at 4°C (△——△). Porcine insulin formulations (40 IU/ml, methylparaben 0.1%, NaCl 0.7%, sodium acetate 10 mM) were stored for 5 1/2 years at 4°C (▲——▲). Bovine rhombohedral insulin crystals (40 IU/ml, phenol 0.2%, NaCl 0.7%, Zn^{2+} 1.3 mM corresponding to approximately 30 Zn per hexamer) were stored for 2 years at 25°C and analyzed for formation of deamidation (○——○) and split A8–A9 products (○ - - - ○). Neutral solutions of porcine insulin (40 IU/ml, methylparaben 0.1%, NaCl 0.7%, sodium phosphate 20 mM) were stored for 4 months at 37°C (●——●).

Degradation products were estimated by disc electrophoresis and densitometric scanning [1]. The neutral solutions showed an approximately 3/1 ratio of B3 isoAsp/Asp derivatives in the pH range 6.8 to 8.

Similar pH profiles were obtained under other storage conditions with alternative species and formulations of insulin.

same rate as in a solution of insulin with the same pH (unpublished observation).

The pH-rate profiles in a broader pH-interval for four different insulin formulations are illustrated in Fig. 3. Deamidation at A21 decreases with increasing pH and becomes virtually undetectable above pH 6. Instead increasing formation of the B3 desamido products (in dissolved and amorphous insulin) or the A8–A9 split product (in certain rhombohedral crystals) can be observed with an increase in pH. Minimal overall hydrolysis takes place at around pH 6.

Over the past three decades, many reports have appeared on the deamidation of, mostly, oligopeptides at neutral pH but only a few of these investigations have addressed the influence of pH on hydrolytic degradation. Our observation that the rate of deamidation around neutrality increases slightly with pH, is in agreement with the findings of others [14, 16, 24, 25, 36]. Capasso *et al.* [36] examined the rate of the individual processes (cyclization+imide hydrolysis) in deamidation of asparaginyl tripeptides and found the rate constants of the formation of the cyclic imide (the rate-determining step in the deamidation reaction) to be approximately 6 times higher at pH 8 than at pH 6.4.

The somewhat smaller difference seen for deamidation of insulin in the same pH interval (Fig. 3) may be attributed to the probably dominating influence of conformational factors on the formation of the intermediate imide which is rate-determining in the deamidation process [37]. It is also noteworthy that the yield of isopeptide relative to normal peptide was relatively constant for insulin in this pH interval (Fig. 3). This is in agreement with studies on the hydrolysis of tri- and hexapeptide succinimides, in which only slight increases in the ratio were observed from pH 6 to 7.5 [24, 36].

The hydrolytic cleavage of the peptide linkage A8–A9 in rhombohedral crystals requires the presence of additional free zinc ions. Thus, no cleavage takes place in the rhombohedral crystals in Biphasic Insulin (Rapitard[R]) containing only four structurally bound zinc ions per hexamer. The cleavage probably arises from catalytic effects of a zinc ion and functional groups within and between hexamers in the rhombohedral crystal resulting in a metalloproteinase-like hydrolysis of the peptide chain [10]. Two His[B5] residues, one from each hexamer, are in proximity to the A8 and A9 residues [35] and coordinated to the zinc ion [27], wich is supposed to activate a water molecule for nucleophilic attack on the carbonyl carbon of the scissile bond [38]. Our observation that the hydrolytic cleavage decreases substantially from pH 7.8 to 6.5 probably reflects protonation of the His residues, which will prevent the zinc coordination necessary for the autocatalytic effect. This pH dependence also explains why the formation of the split product during storage of Insulin Zinc Suspensions initially proceeds relatively quickly, after which it slows down and eventually stops [1]. This extraordinary time profile can be ascribed to the decrease of pH seen during storage of the IZS preparations [7].

Polymerization reactions

The formation of HMWT products was earlier found to be substantially more pronounced in acid as compared to neutral preparations [2]. The formation of HMWT products (mainly CID) as a function of pH is illustrated in Fig. 4. In sharp contrast to the deamidation reactions, the formation of these products decreases with falling pH in the acid range, and at pH 1.5 they are formed at a very low rate. As CID formation is an intra-hexamer reaction, this pH profile reflects the increasing dissociation of hexamers into dimers and monomers [10]. HMWT reveals a maximum at pH 4–4.5 and a minimum at neutral reaction from pH 6.5 to 8. As exemplified for amorphously precipitated insulin (IZS, amorphous), the main products formed below pH 7 in all types of preparation are CIDs with consecutive formation of covalent trimers (Fig. 5). However, at pH 7 to 8, formation of covalent oligo- and polymers (mainly due to disulfide interchange reactions) dominates in this type of preparation when stored at temperatures $\geq 25°C$. In contrast,

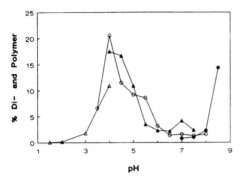

Fig. 4. *Influence of pH on the formation of covalent insulin di- and polymers [2].*
Acid solutions of porcine insulin (40 IU/ml, methylparaben 0.1%, NaCl 0.7%) were stored for 10 days at 37°C (△—△). Bovine rhombohedral insulin crystals (40 IU/ml, phenol 0.2%, NaCl 0.7%, Zn2+ 1.3 mM corresponding to approximately 30 Zn per hexamer) were stored for 1 year at 25°C (○—○). Porcine insulin was formulated as amorphous suspension (40 IU/ml, methylparaben 0.1%, NaCl 0.7%, Zn²⁺ 1.3 mM corresponding to approximately 30 Zn per insulin hexamer) and stored for 6 months at 25°C (▲—▲). Solutions of porcine insulin (40 IU/ml, methylparaben 0.1%, NaCl 0.7%) were stored for 6 months at 25°C (●—●).

Similar pH profiles were obtained under other storage conditions with alternative species and formulations of insulin.

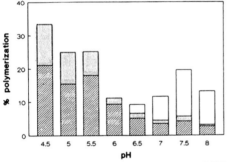

Fig. 5. *Effect of pH on the formation of the individual HMWT products in amorphous suspensions of insulin.*
Porcine insulin (40 IU/ml, methylparaben 0.1%, NaCl 0.7%, Zn²⁺ 1.3 mM corresponding to approximately 30 zinc atoms per insulin hexamer) was formulated as an amorphous suspension and stored for 3 months at 37°C. CID product: hatched bars; Covalent insulin trimers: dotted bars; Covalent insulin oligo- and polymers: open bars.

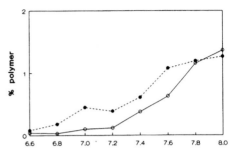

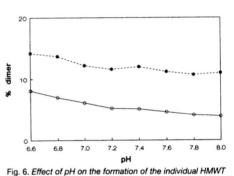

Fig. 6. *Effect of pH on the formation of the individual HMWT products in solutions of insulin around neutrality.*
Porcine insulin solutions (40 IU/ml) containing 0.1% methylparaben and 0.7% NaCl (○—○), or 0.2% phenol and 1.6% glycerol (●--- ●) were stored for 5 months at 37°C.

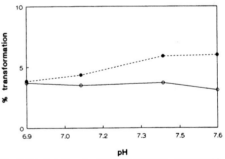

Fig. 7. *Effect of pH on the formation of CID (○—○) and CIPP (●--- ●) in Isophane (NPH) insulin.*
Porcine insulin was formulated as NPH (40 IU/ml) and stored for 4 months at 37°C. To obtain the isophane ratio between protamine and insulin [7], the protamine content per g of insulin was increased from 86 mg at pH 6.9 to 100 mg protamine at pH 7.6 corresponding to approximately 0.7 and 0.8 mol protamine per insulin hexamer, respectively.

in rhombohedral insulin crystals (IZS, crystalline), formation of such polymerization products is not seen [2].

The HMWT products formed in two different formulations of neutral insulin solutions as a function of pH around neutrality are shown in Fig. 6. A slight tendency to reduced CID formation with increasing pH from 6.6 to 8 is observed in both formulations, whereas increasing pH results in a significant increase in the formation of covalent oligo- and polymers, in particular at pH above 7.3.

Table 7. Formation of insulin transformation products (ITP) in Neutral Regular formulations. Dependence of pH and composition.

ITP Product[a]	Formulation[b]	pH				
		7.4	8.0	8.5	9.0	9.5
LMWT	I	0	0	1.1	4.4	7.5
	II	0	0	0.5	1.6	8.9
CID	I	0.8	1.0	1.3	1.9	3.4
	II	0.7	0.7	0.8	2.4	3.5
polymer	I	0	0	1.0	12.5	38.0
	II	0	0	0	1.5	24.2
Total	I	0.8	1.3	3.4	18.8	48.9
transformation	II	0.7	0.7	1.3	5.5	36.6

The figures are the fractions (%) formed after storage for 6 months at 25°C as determined by size exclusion chromatography.
[a] LMWT=Lower molecular weight transformation, i.e. eluting after insulin from the chromatographic column. CID=Covalent insulin dimer.
[b] Regular I was formulated with methylparaben (0.1%) and NaCl (0.7%), II with phenol (0.2%) and glycerol (1.6%).

In the isophane (NPH) preparation, CID formation decreases only slightly in the pH interval 6.9 to 7.6, whereas formation of CIPP increases with pH (Fig. 7). This latter pH trend may be attributed to the increasing content of protamine necessary to obtain the isophane ratio [7] at higher pH values.

A substantial increase in the formation of HMWT products takes place from pH 8.0 to 8.5 (Fig. 4). As can be seen in Table 7, this accelerated formation under mild alkaline conditions is mainly due to the enhanced formation of covalent oligo- and polymers, probably arising as a result of disulfide interactions, as also indicated by the concomitant appearance of lower molecular weight degradation products. These are most likely insulin A- and B-chains originating from disulphide lysis [10].

Conclusions

Auxiliary substances and pH have a profound effect on the chemical stability of insulin in pharmaceutical formulation. The pattern is complex but a common factor both in hydrolysis and intermolecular cross-linking reactions seems to be an influence of excipients on the local conformational structure around the reacting amino acid residues. Some of the reactions are catalytically assisted by insulin functional groups in charged or uncharged form. Therefore, pH also has a complicated influence on the chemical stability since, in addition to its charge effects on insulin and a potential impact on the reaction rate *per se*, it affects the folding and association of the insulin molecules. Thus, a structurereactivity relationship is apparently a main determinant for the chemical transformation of insulin. Optimal over-all stability is observed in the pH range 6–7, which interestingly covers the pH value at which insulin is crystallized

and stored in the pancreatic β-cell [27]. Also today's neutral insulin preparations are formulated at near-optimal pH values.

Acknowledgements

The authors wish to acknowledge the skillful technical assistance of Lene Grønlund Andersen, Helle Irene Arrøe, Lene Bramsen, Lise Frank, Jessie Frederiksen, Lone Jørgensen, Dorte Karkov, Eva Bøg Kristensen and Jette Laulund. We also wish to thank Dr. Svend Havelund for help and advice with the HPLC analyses.

References

1. Brange J., Langkjær L., Havelund S. and Vølund A. (1992) Chemical stability of insulin: 1. Hydrolytic degradation during storage of pharmaceutical preparations. *Pharm. Res. 9*, 715–726
2. Brange J., Havelund S. and Hougaard P. (1992) Chemical stability of insulin: 2. Formation of higher molecular weight transformation products during storage of pharmaceutical preparations. *Pharm. Res. 9*, 727–734
3. Sundby F. (1962) Separation and characterization of acid-induced insulin transformation products by paper electrophoresis in 7 M urea. *J. Biol. Chem. 237*, 3406–3411
4. Brange J., Langkjaer L., Havelund S. and Sørensen E. (1983) Chemical stability of insulin: Neutral insulin solutions. *Diabetologia 25*, 193 (abstract)
5. Helbig H.-J. *Insulindimere aus der b-Komponente von Insulinpräparationen.* Diss., Rheinisch-Westfälische Technische Hochschule, Aachen 1976
6. Brange J., Langkjaer L., Havelund S. and Sørensen E. (1984) Chemical stability of insulin: formation of covalent insulin dimers and other higher molecular weight transformation products in intermediate and long-acting insulin preparations. *Diabetologia 27*, 259A–260A (abstract)
7. Brange J., Skelbaek-Pedersen B., Langkjaer L., Damgaard U., Ege H., Havelund S., Heding L. G., Jørgensen K. H., Lykkeberg J., Markussen J., Pingel M. and Rasmussen E. (1987) *Galenics of Insulin: The Physico-chemical and Pharmaceutical Aspects of Insulin and Insulin Preparations.* Springer-Verlag, Berlin, Heidelberg, New York, London, Paris, Tokyo
8. Wollmer A., Rannefeld B., Johansen B. R., Hejnaes K. R., Balschmidt P. and Hansen F. B. (1987) Phenol-promoted structural transformation of insulin in solution. *Biol. Chem. Hoppe-Seyler 368*, 903–911
9. Derewenda U., Derewenda Z., Dodson E., Dodson G. G., Reynolds C. D., Smith G. D., Sparks C. and Swenson D. (1989) Phenol stabilizes more helix in a new symmetrical zinc insulin hexamer. *Nature 338*, 594–596
10. Brange J. (1992) Chemical stability of insulin: 4. Mechanisms and kinetics of chemical transformations in pharmaceutical formulation. *Acta Pharm. Nord.* in press
11. McGraw S. E., Craik D. J. and Lindenbaum S. (1990) Testing of insulin hexamer-stabilizing ligands using theoretical binding, microcalorimetry, and nuclear magnetic resonance (NMR) line broadening techniques. *Pharm. Res. 7*, 600–605
12. McGraw S. E. and Lindenbaum S. (1990) The use of microcalorimetry to measure thermodynamic parameters of the binding of ligands to insulin. *Pharm. Res. 7*, 606–611
13. McKerrow J. H. and Robinson A. B. (1971) Deamidation of asparaginyl residues as a hazard in experimental protein and peptide procedures. *Anal. Biochem. 42*, 565–568
14. Scotchler J. W. and Robinson A. B. (1974) Deamidation of glutaminyl residues: Dependence on pH, temperature, and ionic strength. *Anal. Biochem. 59*, 319–322

15. Bhatt N. P., Patel K. and Borchardt R. T. (1990) Chemical pathways of peptide degradation. I. Deamidation of adrenocorticotropic hormone. *Pharm. Res. 7*, 593–599

16. Flatmark T. (1966) On the heterogeneity of beef heart Cytochrome C. III. A kinetic study of the non-enzymic deamidation of the main subfractions (Cy I–Cy III). *Acta Chem. Scand. 20*, 1487–1496

17. Tyler-Cross R. and Schirch V. (1991) Effects of amino acid sequence, buffers and ionic strength on the rate and mechanism of deamidation of asparagine residues in small peptides. *J. Biol. Chem. 266*, 22549–22556

18. Yüksel K. Ü. and Gracy R. W. (1986) *In vitro* deamidation of human triosephosphate isomerase. *Arch. Biochem. Biophys. 248*, 452–459

19. Brange J., Havelund S., Hansen P., Langkjaer L., Sørensen E. and Hildebrandt P. (1982) Formulation of physically stable neutral insulin solutions for continuous infusion by delivery systems. In: Gueriguian J. L., Bransome E. D., Outschoorn A. S. (eds). *Hormone Drugs*, Rockville, MD, US Pharmacopoeial Convention, pp 96–105

20. Bello J. and Bello H. R. (1976) Chemical modification and crosslinking of proteins by impurities in glycerol. *Arch. Biochem. Biophys. 172*, 608–610

21. Acharya A. S. and Manning J. M. (1983) Reaction of glycolaldehyde with proteins: Latent crosslinking potential of α-hydroxyaldehydes. *Proc. Natl. Acad. Sci. USA 80*, 3590–3594

22. Brange J. and Havelund S. (1983) Insulin pumps and insulin quality – requirements and problems. *Acta Med. Scand. Suppl. 671*, 135–138

23. Shifrin S. and Parrott C. L. (1975) Influence of glycerol and other polyhydric alcohols on the quaternary structure of an oligomeric protein. *Arch. Biochem. Biophys. 166*, 426–432

24. Patel K. and Borchardt R. T. (1990) Chemical pathways of peptide degradation. II. Kinetics of deamidation of an asparaginyl residue in a model hexapeptide. *Pharm. Res. 7*, 703–711

25. Lura R. and Schirch V. (1988) Role of peptide conformation in the rate and mechanism of deamidation of asparaginyl residues. *Biochemistry 27*, 7671–7677

26. Brange J., Havelund S., Hommel E., Sørensen E. and Kühl C. (1986) Neutral insulin solutions physically stabilized by addition of Zn^{2+}. *Diabetic Med. 3*, 532–536

27. Emdin S. O., Dodson G. G., Cutfield J. M. and Cutfield S. M. (1980) Role of zinc in insulin biosynthesis. Some possible zinc-insulin interactions in the pancreatic B-cell. *Diabetologia 19*, 174–182

28. Brange J., Ribel U., Hansen J. F., Dodson G., Hansen M. T., Havelund S., Melberg S. G., Norris F., Norris K., Snel L., Sørensen A. R. and Voigt H. O. (1988) Monomeric insulins obtained by protein engineering and their medical implications. *Nature 333*, 679–682

29. Hansen J. F. (1991) The self-association of zinc-free human insulin and insulin analogue B13-glutamine. *Biophys. Chem. 39*, 107–110

30. Brange J., Hallund O. and Sørensen E. (1992) Chemical stability of insulin: 5. Isolation, characterization and identification of insulin transformation products. *Acta Pharm. Nord.* submitted

31. Brange J., Langkjaer L., Havelund S. and Sørensen E. (1985) Chemical stability of insulin: formation of desamido insulins and other hydrolytic products in intermediate- and long-acting insulin preparations. *Diabetes Res. Clin. Pract.* (suppl. 1):67 (abstract)

32. Leach S. J. and Lindley H. (1953) The kinetics of hydrolysis of the amide group in proteins and peptides. Part 2. Acid hydrolysis of glycyl- and l-leucyl-l-asparagine. *Trans. Faraday Soc. 49*, 921–925

33. Carpenter F. H. (1966) Relationship of structure to biological activity of insulin as revealed by degradative studies. *Am. J. Med. 40*, 750–758

34. Kirby A. J. and Lancaster P. W. (1972) Structure and efficiency in intramolecular and enzymic catalysis. Catalysis of amide hydrolysis by the carboxy-group of substituted maleamic acids. *J. Chem. Soc. Perkin II* 1206–1214

35. Baker E. N., Blundell T. L., Cutfield J. F., Cutfield S. M., Dodson E. J., Dodson G. G., Hodgkin D. M. C., Hubbard R. E., Isaacs N. W., Reynolds C. D., Sakabe K., Sakabe N. and Vijayan N. M. (1988) The structure of 2Zn pig insulin crystals at 1.5 Å resolution. *Phil. Trans. R. Soc. 319*. 369–456

36. Capasso S., Mazzarella L., Sica F. and Zagari A. (1989) Deamidation via cyclic imide in a sparaginyl peptides. *Peptide Research 2*, 195–200

37. Clarke S. (1987) Propensity for spontaneous succinimide formation from aspartyl and asparaginyl residues in cellular proteins. *Int. J. Peptide Protein Res. 30*, 808–821

38. Hangauer D. G., Monzingo A. F. and Matthews B. W. (1984) An interactive computer graphics study of thermolysin-catalyzed peptide cleavage and inhibition by N-carboxymethyl dipeptides. *Biochemistry 23*, 5730–5741

Received March 18, 1992.
Modified version accepted April 30, 1992.

Reproduced from *Acta Pharmaceutica Nordica*, 4(4):209–222,
1992. Copyright Swedish Pharmaceutical Society. With permission.

Chemical stability of insulin

4. Mechanisms and kinetics of chemical transformations in pharmaceutical formulation

Jens Brange

Novo Research Institute, Novo Alle, DK-2880 Bagsværd, Denmark

Insulin decomposes by a multitude of chemical reactions [1–3]. It deamidates at two different residues by
entirely different mechanisms. In acid, deamidation at Asn ^{A21} is intramolecularly catalyzed by the protonated C-terminal, whereas above pH 6 an intermediate imide formation at residue Asn^{B3} leads to isoAsp
and Asp derivatives. The imide formation requires a large rotation around the α-carbon/peptide carbonyl
carbon bond at B3, corresponding to a 10 Å movement of the B-chain N-terminal. The main determinant
for the rate of B3 deamidation, as well as for the ratio between the two products formed, is the local conformational structure, which is highly influenced by various excipients and the physical state of the insulin.
An amazing thermolysin-like, autoproteolytic cleavage of the A-chain takes place in rhombohedral insulin
crystals, mediated by a concerted catalytic action by several, inter-hexameric functional groups and Zn^{2+}.
Intermolecular, covalent cross-linking of insulin molecules occurs via several mechanisms. The most prominent type of mechanism is aminolysis by the N-terminals, leading to isopeptide linkages with the A-chain
side-chain amides of residues Gln^{A15}, Asn^{A18} and Asn^{A21}. The same type of reaction also leads to covalent
cross-linking of the N-terminal in protamine with insulin. Disulfide exchange reactions, initiated by lysis of
the A7–B7 disulfide bridge, lead mainly to formation of covalent oligo- and polymers. Activation energy
(E_a) for the neutral deamidation and the aminolysis reactions was found to be 80 and 119 KJ/mol, respectively.

In three previous articles in this series, the chemical
stability of insulin was studied in quantitative terms as
a function of various factors relevant for pharmaceutical
formulation [1–3]. A number of different hydrolysis and
covalent higher molecular weight transformation
(HMWT) products have been identified [4]. The main
product in acid medium is monodesamido-(A21)-insu-
lin. In slightly alkaline to slightly acid medium, the transformation products include, dependent on the formulation and actual pH, monodesamido-insulins (Asp^{B3}-
insulin and isoAsp^{B3}-insulin), insulin with a peptide
bond cleavage between residue A8 and A9, and several
different covalent insulin dimers (CID) and polymers.
When protamine is present in the formulation, intermolecular reactions involving the N-terminal of protamine lead to covalent insulin protamine products
(CIPP). In certain formulations at alkaline pH, formation of covalent oligo- and polymers can be observed as
a result of disulfide exchange reactions. Fig. 1 shows the
different sites implicated in the various degradation
reactions.

In the present communication, the kinetics and
mechanisms of the chemical processes leading to deterioration of insulin in therapeutical formulations are
further investigated and discussed.

Experimental

Materials

Insulins used for the studies were monocomponent (MC) insulin of different species (porcine, bovine and human). Potency:
28 IU/mg (dry weight) corresponding to 1.68×10^8 IU/mol. Zn^{2+}

content: 0.4% (w/w of insulin) corresponding to approximately
2 Zn^{2+} per insulin hexamer. Insulin : purity > 99% by reversed-
phase (RP) HPLC. Monodesamido-(A21)-insulin (porcine)
was prepared from MC-insulin by hydrolysis in diluted HCl
(pH 2.5) for 3 months at 25°C. It was separated from remaining
insulin by anion chromatography on QAE Sephadex A-25 and
isolated as described elsewhere [4]. Chemicals were either official (Ph. Eur. or B.P.) or analytical grade.

Analytical procedures

Preparation, storage and isolation of samples for analytical
measurements were performed as described earlier [1]. The
content of covalent HMWT products was estimated by high
performance size exclusion chromatography as described earlier [2].

Molecular modelings were performed by computer graphics
using the Quanta program (Molecular Simulations, Inc. Sun-
nyvale, California).

Results and discussion

Mechanisms

Deamidation

Acid medium: It has long been realized that asparaginyl
peptides are deamidated by acid hydrolysis with greater
ease than the free asparagine [5]. The particular lability
of insulin Asn^{A21} with respect to deamidation can be
ascribed to its position as a C-terminal residue. Leach
and Lindley [6] verified the greater susceptibility in acid
of the side-chain amide of Asn when incorporated in a
peptide, and in investigations on leucyl- and glycylaspa-
ragine dipeptides they showed the rate of deamidation

to increase steeply from pH 3.5 to 2, reaching an essentially constant value below pH 2 [7]. They suggested a mechanism involving a proton transfer from the unionized C-terminal α-COOH group facilitated by a preceding H-bond between the carboxyl hydrogen and the amide nitrogen. In studies on the deamidation of succinamic acids, it was later proposed that the carboxylic acid plays a dual role by attacking the carbonyl carbon atom of the amide, and, simultaneously, donating a proton to the departing ammonia molecule, with formation of a cyclic anhydride [8]. Subsequently, deamidation of insulin in acid medium was proposed to proceed by this mechanism [9, 10], and such a reaction pathway has now been widely recognized as the principal mechanism of the highly efficient intramolecular catalysis of amide hydrolysis by the carboxy-group [11–17]. After proton transfer to the amide group, nucleophilic attack by the carboxylate function forms the tetrahedral intermediate [14] which, after transfer of the proton from the hydroxyl to the nitrogen, breaks down to the anhydride by cleavage of the C-N bond, the rate determining step [15, 17]. Subsequently, the anhydride is readily hydrolyzed by general acid catalysis. Our results [1, 3] are consistent with such a mechanism (Scheme 1). When the α-carboxyl group becomes essentially fully protonated at pH 2–3, constant rate of deamidation would be expected with increasing acidity [7, 13]. The additional deamidation of insulin observed from pH 1 to 0.3 [18] and from pH 2 to 1.5 [3] can, however, be accounted for by further deamidation by direct hydronium ion catalyzed amide hydrolysis, not only of the A21 amide but also of the other five amide groups in insulin, as actually observed. The possibility that other functional groups within the insulin monomer or dimer might be able to approach the A21 group and form hydrogen bonds to the amide, and thereby catalytically assist in the deamidation of A21 [19], adds to the complexity of this reaction.

Neutral medium. Deamidation at neutral and alkaline pHs of peptides and proteins containing Asn residues is generally accepted as primarily proceeding through a cyclic imide intermediate formed by the intramolecular attack of the peptide bond nitrogen of the succeeding residue on the side-chain carbonyl carbon of the Asn residue (Scheme 2). This intramolecular imide is subsequently hydrolyzed by nucleophilic attack by water or hydroxide ions into a mixture of two different desamido products in which the polypeptide backbone is linked via an α-carboxyl linkage (Asp-derivative) or via a β-carboxyl linkage (isoAsp-derivative). Evidence for a succinimide deamidation mechanism occurring in proteins has been obtained for porcine adrenocorticotropin [20, 21], seminal ribonuclease [22], mouse epidermal growth factor [23], α-crystallin [24], trypsin [25], bovine calbindin [26], calmodulin [27], somatropin [28], and serine hydroxymethyltransferase [29]. Our studies [1, 3, 4] strongly indicate that insulin deamidation at B3 Asn proceeds via the same pathway. The initial nucleophilic attack of the main-chain peptide nitrogen on the carbonyl carbon of the side-chain is only possible if these atoms are able to align properly for this reaction. This depends on the side-chain bulkiness of the residue on the C-terminal side of the asparaginyl residue [30–34] as well as on the three-dimensional conformation and flexibility around the Asn residue [19, 25, 35–37]. Optimal conformation for imide formation occurs when the dihe-

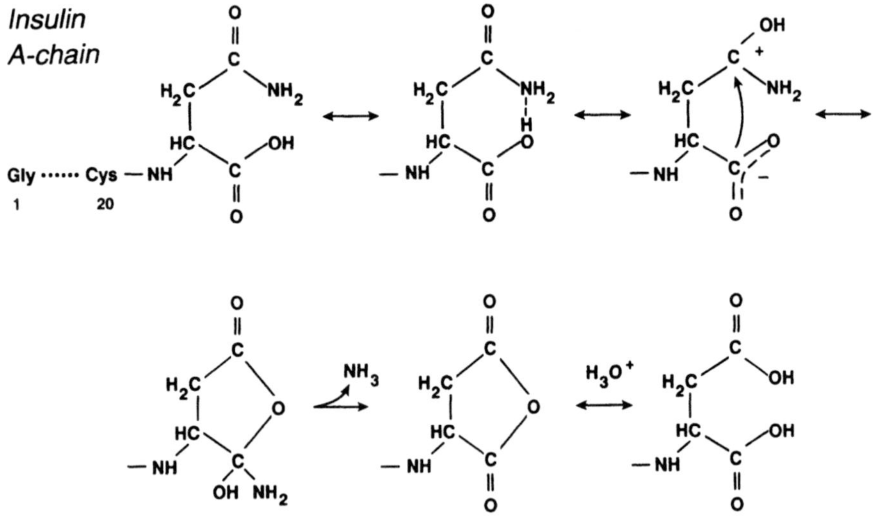

Scheme 1

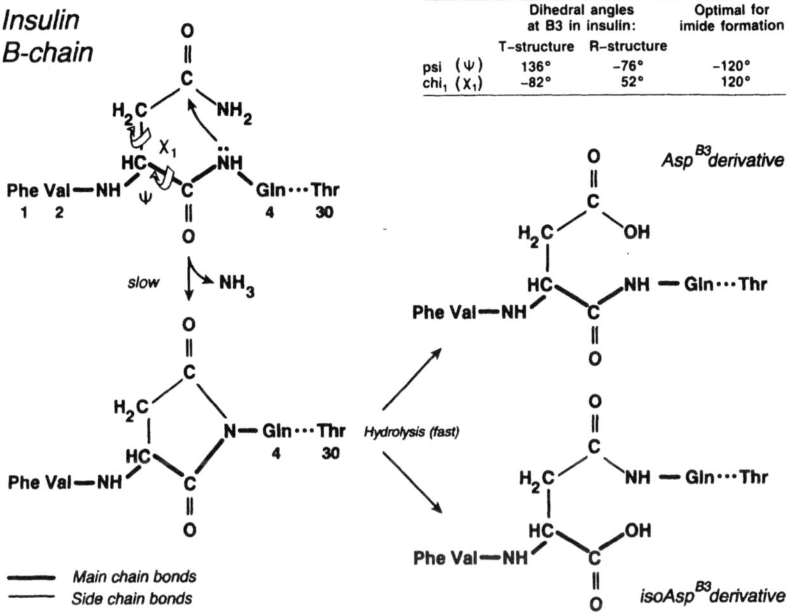

Insulin B-chain

	Dihedral angles at B3 in insulin:		Optimal for imide formation
	T-structure	R-structure	
psi (ψ)	136°	-76°	-120°
chi$_1$ (χ_1)	-82°	52°	120°

Phe Val—NH $\cdots$ C $\cdots$ Gln $\cdots$ Thr
1   2   4   30

slow $\rightarrow$ NH$_3$

Phe Val—NH $\cdots$ N—Gln $\cdots$ Thr   *Hydrolysis (fast)*
                        4   30

Asp^{B3} derivative

Phe Val—NH $\cdots$ NH—Gln $\cdots$ Thr

Phe Val—NH $\cdots$ NH—Gln $\cdots$ Thr

isoAsp^{B3} derivative

——— Main chain bonds
——— Side chain bonds

Scheme 2

dral torsion angles psi (ψ) (defining the rotation around the α-carbon/peptide carbonyl carbon bond) and chi$_1$ (χ_1) (defining the rotation around the α-carbon/β-carbon bond) are -120° and 120°, respectively [35]. Of the three Asn residues in insulin (Fig. 1), one is at the C-terminal, and therefore not able to form succinimide, and A18 is flanked at the C-terminal side by an inhibitory

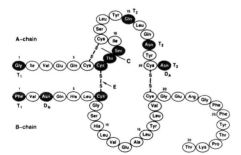

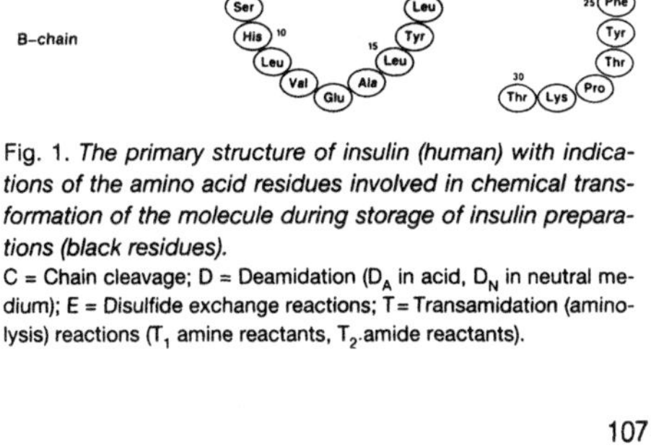

Fig. 1. *The primary structure of insulin (human) with indications of the amino acid residues involved in chemical transformation of the molecule during storage of insulin preparations (black residues).*
C = Chain cleavage; D = Deamidation (D$_A$ in acid, D$_N$ in neutral medium); E = Disulfide exchange reactions; T = Transamidation (aminolysis) reactions (T$_1$ amine reactants, T$_2$ amide reactants).

[30, 34], bulky Tyr. In contrast, the Asn^{B3} is flanked by the relatively less bulky Gln residue. Neither of these two Asn residues has an optimal psi angle, and proper alignment for imide formation requires for both residues a rotation of about 100° around the α-carbon/peptide carbonyl carbon bond (see Scheme 2). However, the B3 residue is on the surface of the hexamer and, perhaps more importantly, the vibrational freedom of its side-chain and main-chain atoms is high as indicated by the crystallographic B values which, for both the main-chain and side-chain, are 2–3 times those of residue A18 [38].

When insulin is in its so-called 2Zn structure (also termed T conformation, see below) the ψ and χ_1 rotations necessary for optimal line-up for succinimide formation at residue B3 are 104° and 158°, respectively. Molecular modeling has shown that such a large change of the dihedral angle ψ at B3, assuming unchanged dihedral angles at other residues, would cause an approximately 10 Å movement of the N-terminal B1 residue (Fig. 2). However, this is possible because the N-terminal residues are on the surface of the insulin hexamer and no steric hindrance applies. In comparison, the A18 residue, being positioned in an α-helix [38] and close to a disulfide bridge, does not have the same possibility for a large change in the dihedral angles.

The 10 Å movement of the B1 residue is actually relatively small when compared with the movement of more

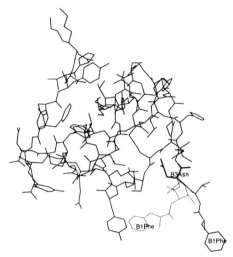

Fig. 2. *The tertiary structure of the insulin monomer in its 2 Zn ("T") conformation shown with the B1–B3 residues in two different positions.*
The normal conformation is drawn with thin lines; the other position corresponds to a rotation of the B3 ψ dihedral angle of 104° (necessary for optimal line-up for succinimide formation at B3) without any other change of dihedral angles. The movement of the Phe^B1 residue is about 10 Å.

than 25 Å of the same residue taking place during the phenol-promoted helix formation at B1–B8 [39]. In this insulin structure (R conformation), the B1–B8 residues have switched into an α-helix which is mainly buried within the hexamer (Fig. 3). Although the B3 ψ dihedral angle in the R-conformation is more favorable for imide formation (Scheme 2), the reduced conformational flexibility in this state is considerably reduced and

makes imide formation less likely. Thus the stabilizing effect of phenol with respect to deamidation [3] is mediated via an influence on insulin conformation.

The sites of succinimide formation and subsequent deamidation in calmodulin also appear to be located in flexible regions of the polypeptide (27, 40). In the case of ribonuclease A, deamidation requires a partial unfolding of the protein to attain the necessary flexibility [41].

It is of interest to note that insulin deamidates in B3 at the same rate whether it is in neutral solution or is precipitated in amorphous form by zinc ions. In rhombohedral insulin crystals, however, the rate of deamidation is reduced [1].

Ratio isoAsp/Asp. The successive, relatively fast progressing, hydrolytic opening of the intermediate succinimide derivative under neutral to alkaline conditions can occur at either the α-carbonyl group (to yield an isoaspartyl residue) or at the β-carbonyl group (to form a normal aspartyl residue) (Scheme 2). The ring opening of the imide is governed by the relative electrophilic character of the two carbonyl groups in the ring which through electron-inductive effect would favor attack at the α-carbonyl group [42]. Model studies on oligopeptides [31, 32, 34, 37, 43–45] have shown that the hydrolytic process generates a mixture of these derivatives with an approximately 3:1 predominance of the isoaspartyl residue (i.e. original Asn transformed to isoAsp with a free α-caboxylate group) relative to the normal peptide.

In neutral solutions of insulin, the formation of the isoAsp derivative also dominates relative to the Asp derivative but the ratio is reduced to 1.9 and 1.4 for solutions containing methylparaben and phenol, respectively [1]. This decreased formation of isoAsp relative to Asp derivative when the Asn residue is part of a protein with a tertiary structure, is in agreement with findings on deamidation of α-crystallin [24] and of serine hydroxymethyltransferase [29] (ratios 1.6 and 1, respectively) whereas a ratio of 3–4 was found in deamidation

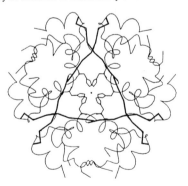 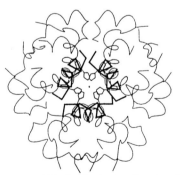

Fig. 3. *The hexamer of insulin shown in two different conformations. To the left is the 2Zn structure (T-conformation), to the right the phenol-promoted structure (R-conformation) with a switch from the extended into the α-helix of the residues B1–B8 (drawn with thick lines) through which the B-chain N-terminal becomes buried in the hexamer.*

of human growth hormone [46] and in NMR studies of r-calbindin [26]. The distribution of the insulin B3-deamidated products is independent of time and temperature [1], and pH around neutrality [3].

In neutral suspensions of amorphously precipitated insulin (i.e. insulin zinc suspension, amorphous) deamidation proceeds at the same rate as in neutral solution, but the hydrolysis of the succinimide intermediate now favors formation of the normal Asp derivative, which accounts for 65% of the total hydrolysis. The same dominance of the Asp derivative over the isoAsp derivative is observed when neutral suspensions of insulin crystals (i.e. insulin zinc suspensions or NPH preparations) undergo deamidation, but total deamidation is much slower [1].

There are several possible explanations for the observed reduction in the isoAsp:Asp ratio when the deamidation takes place in a more or less rigid protein rather than in a conformationally much more flexible peptide without higher order structural elements: 1) Additional deamidation via direct solvent hydrolysis of the side-chain amide; 2) Deamidation of the side-chain amide group assisted by intramolecular catalytic participation of functional groups which, as a result of the three-dimensional structure of the protein, are close to the amide group; 3) Initial ring closure by isoimide formation, in addition to the generation of succinimide, succeeded by hydrolysis of the isoimide into the aspartyl derivative; 4) Reduced accessibility to hydrolysis of the succinimide peptide linkage (isoAsp formation) as compared to the other hydrolyzable bond of the imide due to steric hindrance; 5) Increased susceptibility of the imide β-peptide linkage to hydrolysis due to inductive effect by juxtaposed functional groups in the three-dimensional structure.

The first of these possibilities, direct solvent (or OH^-) mediated hydrolysis of the amide, would be expected to be very slow at neutral reaction. But when the succinimide formation (and the subsequent yield of isoAsp derivative) is substantially reduced, as when insulin is in crystalline state, the relative importance of this pathway for deamidation may increase and account for the reversal of the ratio between isoAsp:Asp. However, the reduction of total deamidation does not apply to the amorphous suspension of insulin with the same low isoAsp:Asp ratio of 0.6:1. Consequently, the increased prevalence of the Asp derivative probably does not originate from intrinsic, direct amide hydrolysis. The reported independence of the ratios on time and temperature [1] also suggests that all deamidation proceeds via the same pathway. This is in agreement with studies on deamidation of asparaginyl-glycyl model peptides, in which no direct side-chain hydrolysis of the primary amide could be detected [43]. It should also be mentioned that during isolation and identification of B3-deamidated insulins, no deamidation of any of the two A-chain asparaginyl residues could be detected [4].

Intramolecular catalytic enhancement of the deamidation of asparaginyl residues into Asp derivatives was proposed as an alternative mechanism for deamidation of proteins by Wright and Robinson [19, 47]. In neutral medium this process was assumed to be general base catalyzed with the participation of particular amino acid residues in proximity to the labile amide side-chain in the secondary and tertiary structure. For deamidation of insulin at Asn^{B3}, a hydrogen bond to O_γ of the nearby Ser^{A12} was suggested to facilitate loss of the amide ammonia-leaving group. Our data on insulin deamidation [1, 3] do not preclude this mechanism to be responsible, at least in part, for the increased fraction of Asp relative to isoAsp derivatives, with increasing stabilization of the tertiary and quaternary structure of insulin. In fact, when phenol is added to a neutral insulin solution, and the isoAsp:Asp ratio decreases from 1.9 to 1.4, the B-chain N-terminal with the B3 residue is embedded into the interior of the hexamer (R-structure) and becomes surrounded by residues able to interact with the amide group (Fig. 3). However, the observation that crystalline insulin suspensions, with insulin in its T-structure (B3 on the surface of the hexamer) and without specific inter-hexameric contacts at B3 [38], exhibit an even lower ratio, contradicts the assumption that this mechanism is solely responsible for the ratio reduction.

Based on earlier work on the formation, properties and reactions of phthal- and succinisoimides [48, 49], an alternative cyclization pathway for Asn residues with formation of a five-membered 4,5-diamino-2-oxalanone ring (isoimide) has been hypothesized [35, 50]. Instead of the nucleophilic attack by the main-chain nitrogen atom on the carbonyl carbon of the side-chain resulting in formation of succinimide, the proposed reaction involves an attack by the peptide carbonyl oxygen on the same carbon atom. Such succinisoimide derivatives are readily hydrolyzed in neutral medium by general acid catalysis into normal aspartyl residues [49]. Optimal attack by the peptide bond oxygen to form an isoimide could be expected when the oxygen is facing the carbonyl carbon of the amide. This is most likely to happen when the dihedral angle ψ between the α-carbon and the carbonyl carbon of the peptide bond approaches $-60°C$. Such a conformation is not very frequent in proteins but might be found in an α-helix [35, 50]. Therefore, when the N-terminal of the insulin B-chain is switched into an α-helix by the influence of phenol, the increasing relative amounts of Asp^{B3} products in deamidation reactions in neutral media (NPH and neutral soluble preparations with phenol preservation) might be accounted for by intermediate isopeptide formation. Indeed, inspection by molecular graphics of the stereogeometry in monoclinic insulin crystals grown in the presence of phenol [39] has revealed that the dihedral angle ψ at B3 is $-50°$ and thus quite close to the optimal value for isoimide formation. Nonetheless, in neutral suspensions of amorphous or crystalline insulin devoid of phenol, i.e. insulin zinc suspensions (IZS), and hence without the helix transformation of the N-terminal, a similar lowering of the ratio is observed.

All cases with reduced ratio share the feature that the B-chain N-terminals have become less accessible, either by being buried within the hexamer (phenol-promoted helix formation) or by further aggregation of the hexameric units (rhombohedral crystals or amorphous precipitate). Stereochemical hindrance has been reported in hydrolysis of succinic anhydride [51] and similar impediments may relate to the imide hydrolysis. This theory would, however, require that the peptide linkage of the imide is better shielded for hydrolytic attack than the other hydrolyzable bond in the imide when this is part of a large peptide with a more fixed tertiary structure.

Normally, in the absence of dominating steric hindrance, the ring opening of the imide occurs mainly at the most electronegative of the two carbonyl groups favoring hydrolysis of the peptide bond, leading to an isoAsp derivative [42]. However, if a hydrogen bond to the former side-chain carbonyl oxygen weakens the carbonyl carbon for nucleophilic attack [52–54], an enhanced hydrolysis of the isopeptide bond and a higher relative yield of the normal Asp derivative might result. Such hydrogen bonding may be realized as a result of the structural changes in the amorphous and crystalline insulin or the switch to α-helix promoted by phenol, and thus offers a plausible explanation of the observed change in the predominance of the individual hydrolytic products.

The hydrolysis of the imide ring is much faster than its formation, wherefore accumulation of the cyclic imide is small. The steady-state concentration of imide in deamidation of hexapeptides at pH 7.4 was calculated to be about 0.2% [31], whereas the relative maximum concentration of imide was observed to be 4–15% of total transformation products in deamidation of tetrapeptides [32]. It is not known whether the analytical methods are able to separate the succinimide B3 derivative from the similarly charged parent insulin but accumulation of the imide is probably too low to be detectable. Recently, isolation of a derivative of methionyl human growth hormone containing an intact cyclic succinimide ring was reported [55] but no quantitative data were given.

A8–A9 chain cleavage

The spontaneous hydrolysis of the peptide chain between residues A8 and A9 in certain insulin preparations [1] is quite unusual, and similar cleavage reactions proceeding at normal temperatures have apparently not been reported previously for any non-enzyme protein. The fact that the cleavage only occurs in rhombohedral insulin crystals in the presence of more than four zinc ions per hexamer suggested an autoproteolytic mechanism requiring zinc ions for the catalytic activity. This theory prompted an analysis of the interactions between

hexamers in the rhombohedral crystals. The A chain loop A8–A10 projects from the surface of the hexamer, and according to Baker et al. [38] the stacking of hexamers in the crystal forces this protruding peptide chain to pack into a gap in the adjacent hexamer surface and thus brings the A8–A9 residues in close proximity to residues in the neighboring hexamer. A proposed mechanism for zinc endopeptidase activity [56] involves nucleophilic attack of a water molecule on the carbonyl carbon of the scissile bond which is activated by a Glu residue acting as a general base. The resulting tetrahedral intermediate is stabilized by His which donates a hydrogen bond to the hydrated peptide. The catalyzing zinc ion, initially coordinated to His, His, Glu and the attacking water molecule, becomes pentacoordinate in the Michaelis complex.

In the interface between hexamers in rhombohedral zinc insulin crystals two B5 His residues from succeeding molecules in different hexamers are in close contacts (4 Å) across the hexamer boundary in proximity to the A8 and A9 residues [38], and they actually form a zinc binding-site within the crystals [57]. In addition, B21 Glu is quite near this hexamer interface domain and, as shown in Fig. 4, its carboxylate group can, by rotation of the side-chain, approach the A8 residue in its own molecule. All the crucial elements for a metalloprotease-mediated attack on the A8 carbonyl carbon (zinc ion, and Glu and His residues) are present, and hence a

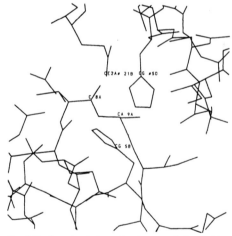

Fig. 4. *The boundary between two hexamers in the stacking of hexamers in rhombohedral insulin crystals.*
The His B5 side-chain (labeled 5D) from one hexamer makes contact with A8 carbonyl carbon (labeled 8A) in the neighboring hexamer and forms, together with His B5 (labeled 5B) from the other hexamer, a zinc binding-site within the crystals (Ref. 57). The side chain of B21 Glu (labeled 21B) is close to this domain and, by rotation of the side-chain, its carboxylate group can approach the A8 residue in its own molecule. Consequently, all elements for a metalloprotease-mediated attack on the A8 carbonyl carbon (zinc ion, and Glu and His residues) are present in the hexamer interface.

mechanism involving a thermolysin-like protease activity is proposed for this reaction. The carboxyl group of B21 Glu can apparently move into a position where it can act as a general base and weaken the A8 carbonyl carbon for nucleophilic attack by a water molecule activated by coordination to a zinc atom which is also coordinated to two B5 His. It is likely that the hydroxyl group in the side-chain of A9 Ser will contribute to some extent to weakening the carbonyl carbon.

The rate of formation of the A8–A9 split product was found to increase in the order human < porcine < bovine insulin [1]. The difference between bovine and porcine insulin might be explained by different A8 residues (Ala and Thr, respectively) but is more likely due to a closer approach between stacking hexamers in bovine insulin crystals. In porcine insulin, the extra methyl group in the A10 residue (Ile), as compared to the respective bovine residue (Val), hinders the same tight packing of the hexamers as in bovine insulin. Although the difference in this distance is only approx. 0.3 Å, this might very well account for the more optimal alignment of the residues involved in the catalytic events and the resulting 4–6 times higher rate constants. The slight difference in the rate of cleavage between porcine and human insulin, with the same primary structure of their A-chains and essentially the same crystal structure as the animal insulins [58], can only be explained by minor conformational differences in the packing of hexamers in the rhombohedral crystal.

A number of metallo-endoproteases, including the most extensively studied metallo-protease, thermolysin, have pH optimum near neutrality [59]. The observation that the split product formation decreases dramatically from pH 7.5 to pH 6.5 [3], probably reflecting the protonation of the His imidazole group which will prevent the Zn coordination necessary for the enzymatic process, supports the theory that the cleavage is an autoproteolytic process.

CID formation

In systematic studies on covalent insulin dimers isolated from crude insulin crystals, Helbig [60] showed that the main product is formed by a intermolecular reaction of the B1 N-terminal amine group with the A21 carboxamide group (A-B dimer). To a minor extent, a link between the N-terminal A-chain and the A21 group was also identified (A-A dimer). A similar intramolecular nucleophilic displacement of an asparaginyl side-chain amide by the amino terminus, involving formation of a seven membered cyclic amide, has been described for a tetrapeptide [37]. In aminolysis of amides, an increasing rate of reaction with the acidity of the medium, reaching an essentially constant value below pH 3, has been observed [61]. This is in agreement with our finding that dimer formation increases substantially with acidity of the medium from pH 7 to 4 [3].

The intermolecular chemical reaction leading to insulin dimer formation seems to take place between insulin molecules in the insulin hexamer [2], the common unit in solutions, as well as in amorphous or crystalline suspensions from pH 4 to 8 [62]. Within the dimeric association units of hexameric insulin, the distances from the B-chain amino terminal to A21 in different molecules are approx. 30 Å (distance through the center of the unit), whereas the similar inter-dimer contacts are about 14 Å (along the surface of the hexamer). The corresponding inter- and intra-dimer distances from the A-chain N-terminal are 33 and 15 Å, respectively, making an intra-dimer approach of this sort possible. However, the flexibility of the A-chain N-terminal is much smaller than that of the N-terminal B-chain [38] which probably explains why a 2:1 predominance of A-B versus A-A dimers was found in both crystalline and in amorphous pharmaceutical suspensions [4]. The finding that dimer formation in solutions of insulin is independent of the concentration of hexameric insulin [2] strongly indicates that the reactions between the N-terminals and A21 in different molecules mainly takes place between different monomers within the hexamer. In order to make the aminolysis reaction possible, an approximately 10 Å approach between the involved terminals in different monomers would be necessary. As the reactants are on the surface of the hexamer, movements of this size are conceivable when the hexamers are in solution although more restrained mobility would apply when the hexamers are incorporated in a crystal. However, major conformational rearrangement would be more likely at the surface as compared to the interior of the crystals. To address this question, insulin crystals of different sizes, formulated as the IZS type preparation, were tested. As 10 and 100 micron crystals showed the same rate of CID formation, it can be concluded that the reaction occurs to the same extent in the interior as at the surface of the crystal. In the crystalline preparations, the CID formation therefore leads to bridging of the individual monomers within the hexamer in the crystal lattice. Such crosslinking of the individual molecules in the crystals of IZS (crystalline), heat treated at a pH (5.5) with substantially increased rate of CID formation [3], is probably the reason for the "thermic effect" resulting in extreme retardation of the timing of action [63].

The intermolecular reactions within the crystal lattice would dictate quite a sizeable spatial mobility within the individual hexamers in the crystals but evidence for such an intrinsic plasticity of crystalline proteins has recently been emphasized [64], and the N-terminal insulin B-chain in particular has revealed its immense capacity for large conformational rearrangements [39, 65] even within an existing crystal lattice [65].

In all pharmaceutical neutral solutions as well as in amorphous and crystalline suspensions, formation of at least 5–6 different covalent dimers is observed by RP-HPLC, namely 3–4 major components (each ≥ 10% of total dimer formation) and 2–3 minor components [4].

Table 1. *Formation of covalent HMWT products in different insulins.*

Insulin	Product formed	Temperature (°C)					
		37			45		
		1 week	5 weeks	9 weeks	1 week	2 weeks	5 weeks
Monodesamido-	CID	< 0.1	0.3	0.7	0.3	0.7	3.2
(A 21)-insulin	Polymer	< 0.1	0.7	1.2	1.8	no data	18.3
(porcine)	total HMWT	< 0.2	1.0	1.9	2.1		21.5
Porcine	CID	0.1	0.7	1.3	0.5	1.1	2.4
insulin	Polymer	< 0.1	< 0.1	< 0.1	< 0.1	< 0.1	0.5
	total HMWT	~ 0.1	~ 0.7	1.3	~ 0.5	1.1	2.9

The figures are the percentage formed of the individual products. The insulin solutions (0.24 mM ~ 40 UI/ml), containing two zinc atoms per hexamer, were formulated with methylparaben and NaCl at pH 7.4.

This implies that amides other than Asn^{A21} are involved in the process. Indeed, inspection of the crystal structure actually shows that the amide group of Asn^{A18} is even closer to the B1 amino group (inter-dimer distance 11 Å) and Gln^{A15} is within a 15 Å distance. Although A21 is probably more reactive, due to the possibility of catalytic assistance of the C-terminal carboxyl group, it seems logical that also the two other amido groups can participate in intermolecular aminolysis reactions. Good evidence for involvement of alternative amido groups in CID formation has been obtained by ageing a neutral solution of monodesamido-(A21)-insulin. Despite the fact that the charged A21 side-chain in this derivative is probably unable to react, dimers and polymers are still formed (Table 1). The rate of CID formation in the deamidated insulin is in most cases 40–60% of that of the native insulin.

The pH dependence of the dimerization reaction [3] is in agreement with a proposed mechanism in which the amine base and a proton source (hydronium ion or, if A21 is involved, the protonated carboxyl group) attack the amide bond in concert ([61], Scheme 3). The steep

fall in the rate of covalent dimer formation from pH 4 to 3.5 [3] most likely reflects the dissociation of the hexamer into mainly dimeric units [66], and providing further evidence for CID formation primarily being an inter-dimer reaction occurring within the hexamer. Below pH 2, virtually no covalent dimer formation is observed, probably as a result of increasing dissociation of dimers into monomers, competition from the dominating hydrolysis of Asn^{A21} amido group, or both.

In glycerol-containing preparations, part of the CID fraction might be generated via Schiff base formation by aldehyde impurities followed by Amadori rearrangement and subsequent cross-linking of insulin molecules [2].

CIPP formation

The covalent insulin protamine complex is most likely formed in an aminolysis reaction by the N-terminal amino group of protamine similar to the CID formation. Protamine is rather loosely bound in the NPH crystals, where it mediates interactions between dimers in the

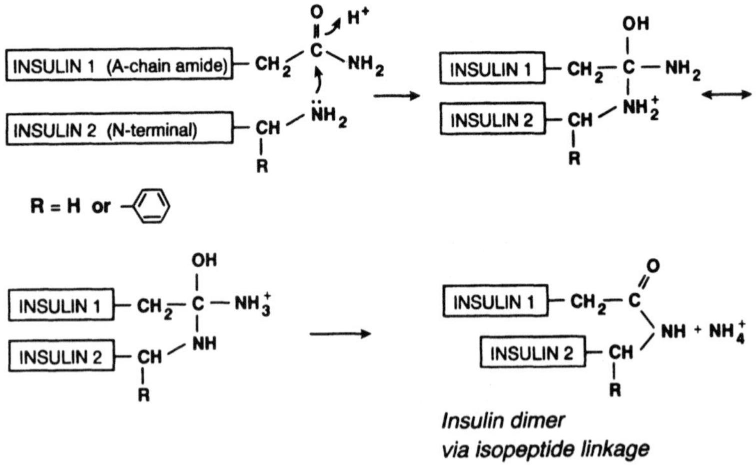

Scheme 3

112

hexamer in which it penetrates the polar central channel. In the interstices between hexamers, it is also involved in hexamer-hexamer contacts but generally exhibits large conformational flexibility [67]. Because of this flexibility of the protamine molecule, its N-terminal amino group has the capacity and possibilities to react with insulin by the same mechanisms as in the CID formation. In accordance with this theory, it has been shown that the CIPP formation is substantially reduced, but not entirely prevented, when the amino group of protamine is blocked (Lykkeberg, personal communication). Hence, the residual amount of CIPP must be explained by alternative reaction pathways. Theoretically, such cross-linking reactions might involve the many arginyl residues in protamine and oxidation products of *m*-cresol that might be able to make condensation products. As in CID formation, aldehyde impurities in glycerol may also be able, via Schiff base formation and Amadori rearrangement, to contribute to cross-linking insulin and protamine.

Formation of covalent insulin oligo- and polymers

Insulin forms in neutral solution and amorphous suspension, in parallel to the formation of CID products, covalent polymerization products [2] and, above pH 8, cleavage into A- and B-chains can also be observed [3]. Such products are the result of disulfide lysis and interchange reactions [4]. Degradation of protein disulfide bonds at high pH values under formation of a variety of products is a well-established phenomenon [68] but the mechanism of the S-S-bond lysis is under dispute [69, 70]. The initial product of the disulfide cleavage is believed to be a persulfide intermediate [71] formed by a β-elimination reaction with the generation of dehydro-

alanine residues ([69], Scheme 4). The persulfide is subsequently decomposed into thiol and sulfur or hydrolyzed to form a sulphenic acid which further decomposes to produce thiol and sulphinic acid [69]. Even traces of thiolate ions are able to initiate disulfide exchange reactions [71–73] by nucleophilic attack on a sulfur atom of a disulfide. Whereas the hydroxyl ion-catalyzed rupture of the S-S-bond requires high alkalinity, the thiolate-induced cleavage proceeds at pH values as low as 8–9 [71]. In studies on the lysis of the disulfide bonds of insulin by sulfhydryl compounds at pH 9, evidence was found that the cleavage proceeded via the β-elimination mechanism with formation of intermediate persulfide [70] and dehydroalanine residues [74]. Whatever the pathway, each reaction leaves a new reactive thiolate ion which is able to undergo fast thiol-disulfide interchange. The dehydroalanine-containing products may also undergo secondary reactions [74], e.g. by condensation with amines (Scheme 4 1.2). It is unclear how the initial disulfide cleavage with formation of a thiolate ion can proceed (temperatures above 25°C) at pH values as low as 7.4 [2]. However, as soon as the first thiolate ion is formed, the chain reaction starts with continuous generation of new thiols able to react with further disulfide residues. As discussed earlier, the initial intermolecular disulfide exchange requires juxtaposition of disulfide bridges from different insulin molecules and is most likely an inter-hexamer reaction [2, 3]. However, as the cleavage of the first disulfide bridge probably causes some unfolding of the molecule, the following interchange reactions are presumably facilitated by exposure of further disulfide residues. Of the three disulfide bridges in insulin, only the inter-chain A7–B7 bridge is near the surface of the folded monomeric molecule, and it is not buried by association of insulin into a hexamer [38].

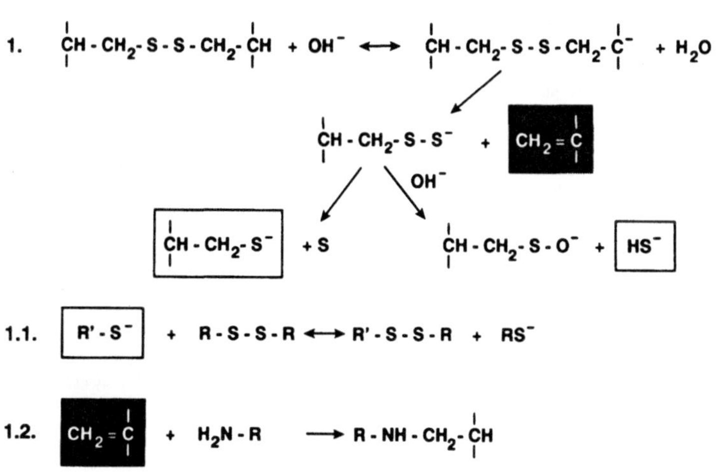

Scheme 4

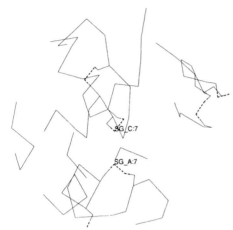

Fig. 5. *The interface between two insulin hexamers which have manually been docked together in order to make the closest possible contact between disulfide bridges (shown with broken lines).*
Two sulfur atoms (A7 and C7) from different A7–B7 bridges are brought within bond-forming distance between the two hexamers.

Molecular modeling has shown that two sulfur atoms from individual hexamers can be brought within bond-forming distance by docking the hexamers (Fig. 5). In neutral formulations, proper inter-hexamer contact for disulfide exchange is possible in dissolved and amorphous preparations but not in crystalline preparations [2].

With increasing pH above pH 8, polymerization due to intermolecular disulfide exchange increases exponentially [3]. This rate enhancement can most likely be attributed to more initial thiolate formation from the cleavage of disulfide (rate-determining step). However, as the charged thiol is the active species (pK about 8.5), the increasing deprotonation of the thiol group may also contribute to the rate acceleration. In addition, dissociation of the insulin hexamer and dimer at increasing pH above 8 [66] provides more favorable conditions for intermolecular contacts.

In accordance with the numerous theoretical possibilities for the formation of different oligo- and polymeric products, a multitude of compounds can be observed by analytical isoelectric focusing on a 10–40 kD fraction from size-exclusion chromatography of an aged amorphous insulin zinc suspension [4].

Kinetics

Insulin deamidation proceeds rapidly in acid formulations by amide hydrolysis at residue Asn[A21] [1, 18]. In a neutral formulation, hydrolysis takes place only at residue Asn[B3] and at a substantially reduced rate compared with the acid formulations [1]. The particular susceptibility to hydrolysis of the C-terminal amide Asn [A21] in

acid medium as compared with the other 2 Asn residues is, as previously discussed, due to intramolecular catalysis by the protonated C-terminal carboxyl group. As the rate-determining step is the formation of the anhydride, the rate of hydrolysis can be expected to be a function of the degree of protonation of the terminal α-carboxyl group. Accordingly, the rate of deamidation of insulin has been shown to increase with decreasing pH in the pH interval 5–1.5 [3].

Deamidation of Asn residues under neutral or alkaline conditions occurs via formation of a cyclic imide intermediate, which is a relatively slow reaction and therefore rate-determining for the entire deamidation reaction [31, 43]. The imide ring is subsequently hydrolyzed relatively fast at either of the two C-N bonds. Due to the relatively slow rate of deamidation of insulin at lower temperatures, and the complexity of the chemical transformation reactions in combination with the propensity of insulin to form non-covalent aggregation products and precipitates at higher temperatures [62, 75], experiments designed to deamidate insulin by 2–3 half-lives were not successful. The deamidation data previously obtained [1] do not allow any definite estimation of the order of reaction but it is reasonable to assume first-order kinetics as found for the deamidation of hexapeptides [30–32] and of proteins [21, 41]. This assumption is supported by the observation that the rate of deamidation is independent of the insulin concentration from 40–400 IU/ml [1].

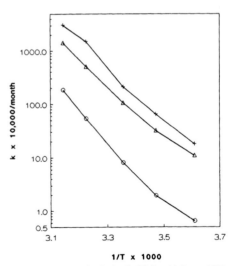

Fig. 6. *Arrhenius plots for the insulin B3 deamidation and CID formation in neutral pharmaceutical solutions based on data from Refs. 1 and 2.*
Deamidation in solutions containing NaCl and methylparaben: + – +; glycerol and phenol: △ – △. CID formation in solution containing NaCl and methylparaben: ○ – ○.

Arrhenius-type plots for the deamidation and covalent dimerization of insulin in neutral pharmaceutical solutions, based on previously published data [1, 2], are shown in Fig. 6. Only within certain temperature intervals can linearity of these plots be observed. The rate of deamidation increases more with temperature than expected from the Arrhenius equation, which probably reflects the increase in conformational freedom around the deamidating B3 residue with increasing temperature. As the intermediate formation of the succinimide ring is the rate-determining step in the transformation reaction, it is conceivable that the overall reaction is facilitated when a higher temperature increases the possibility for the main-chain and side-chain groups to assume the conformation necessary for succinimide formation.

From the linear parts of the slopes in the Arrhenius plots, the activation energy (E_a) for the deamidation reaction is calculated to be 80.3 kJ/mol (19.2 kcal/mol) and 106 kJ/mol (25.3 kcal/mol) in neutral insulin solutions containing NaCl and methylparaben (4–25°C), and glycerol and phenol (25–45°C), respectively. These values are in good agreement with the values 21.7 and 22.5 kcal/mol found under similar conditions by Patel and Borchardt [33], and Geiger and Clarke [31], respectively, for the deamidation of asparaginyl hexapeptides (Asn-Gly sequence). A somewhat lower value (15.2 kcal/mol) has been found for deamidation of reduced, unfolded RNase A at pH 7.2 [41].

Half-lives for the deamidation of insulin in two different neutral solutions are shown in Table 2, together with similar data at 37°C from the literature for deamidation of asparaginyl penta- and hexapeptides. Compared with the most stable peptides, $T_{1/2}$ for insulin, in its most unstable formulation, is only slightly longer than for the peptides, a clear indication of the great flexibility of the B-chain N-terminal segment for attaining the proper alignment for imide formation and subsequent hydrolysis. Against this background, the very

short half-life of less than one day observed for deamidation of bovine seminal ribonuclease [76] is quite remarkable.

In all pharmaceutical preparations, temperature has a profound influence on the rate of formation of hydrolysis as well as HMWT-products. The relative effect of increasing the temperature by 10°C (temperature coefficient Q_{10}) on the formation of B3 deamidation products in the temperature interval 4–25°C was found to be approximately 3 for all formulations, except NPH, in which the coefficient is < 2 [1]. Apparently, the structural stabilization by m-cresol (or phenol) in this type of preparation is equally effective at 4° and 25°C. In comparison, in the formulations with insulin in amorphous or dissolved form, allowing more conformational flexibility in the molecule, imide formation at B3 is facilitated by increasing temperature also for steric reasons. The temperature coefficient for split product (A8–A9) formation is as high as 10, which probably reflects the need for quite sizeable thermal fluctuations and displacements in the three-dimensional structure for the interhexamer catalytic process to take place.

Temperature coefficients Q_{10} for the formation of CID and covalent polymers are shown in Table 3 for different temperature intervals. For CID formation, a tendency to slightly increased Q_{10} with increasing temperature in the interval from 4–25°C can be observed. In all preparations, except the NPH type, an increase in temperature from 25°C to 37°C causes a more dramatic increase in Q_{10}, after which the values again undergo reduction in the interval 37°–45°C. The corresponding temperature coefficients for formation of covalent polymers reach unusually high values whereas the figures for CIPP are more similar to the values for formation of CID. For the covalent di- and polymerization of insulin in neutral solution (containing 0.7% NaCl and 0.1% methylparaben) E_a (15–45°C) is, from the slope of the Arrhenius plot (Fig. 6), calculated to be 118.8 kJ/mol (28.4 kcal/mol). None of the other data sets for HMWT

Table 2. Degradation times (days) for deamidation of insulin and different oligopeptides at pH 7.4.

Compound	Formulation	Temperature (°C)	$T_{1\%}$	$T_{10\%}$	$T_{50\%}$	Reference
Insulin	NaCl (0.7%)	4	171			
	methylparaben (0.1%)	25	14	153		
	acetate (10 mM)	37	2.2	24	150	
	glycerol (1.6%)	4	278			1
	phenol (0.2%)	25	28	299		
		37	6	69	415	
-Asn-Glu-pentapeptide	phosphate, ionic				12	
-Asn-Arg-pentapeptide	strength 0.15				20	79
-Asn-Arg-pentapeptide	TRIS, ionic strength 0.15	37			115	
-Asn-Gly-hexapeptide					1	
-Asn-Leu-hexapeptide	phosphate 0.1 M				70	31
-Asn-Pro-hexapeptide					106	
-Asn-Ala-hexapeptide					20	36
-Asn-Ser-hexapeptide					8	

The insulin data were calculated from rate data [1] assuming first order kinetics.

Table 3. *Effect of temperature on formation of covalent HMWT products in pharmaceutical preparations.*

Preparation[a]	Product	Temperature interval (°C)[b]			
		4–15	15–25	25–37	37–45
Regular I	CID	2.7	3.3	5.9	4.4
	Polymer			2.5	95
Regular II	CID	2.0	3.1	4.6	
IZS amorph.	CID	3.9	4.1	7.3	2.0
	Polymer			16	3.0
IZS cryst.	CID	4.1	6.1	9.5	5.0
NPH,	CID	4.1	3.0	3.7	3.7
40 IU/ml	CIPP	3.2	2.6	4.5	3.8
NPH,	CID	2.7	3.4	4.1	3.4
100 IU/ml	CIPP	2.1	3.3	3.8	3.7

[a] Regular I was formulated with methylparaben and NaCl, Regular II with phenol and glycerol. Abbreviations: IZS: Insulin zinc suspension; NPH: Neutral protamine Hagedorn (Isophane insulin); CID: covalent insulin dimer; CIPP: covalent insulin protamine product.
[b] The figures are the temperature coefficient Q_{10} calculated on the basis of the expression $\log Q_{10} = 10 \times (\log k_2 - \log k_1)/(T_2 - T_1)$, using rate data from ref. 2.

product formation [2] give linear Arrhenius plots. The temperature-dependence of the di- and polymerization reactions varies from one type of preparation to another, probably due to variations in the extent to which an increase in temperature influences the structural flexibility of the insulin molecule in the various formulations. The relatively large increase of Q_{10} around 30°C in most preparations probably reflects a progressive weakening in the interactions within the hexamer, contributing to the structural stability at lower temperatures. The NPH preparation does not exhibit this effect to the same extent, possibly due to an additional stabilizing effect of the phenol (or cresol) [39, 67].

Impact of three-dimensional structure

Insulin is chemically transformed by a multitude of different reactions, some of which are mediated, intra- or intermolecularly, by catalytic participation of insulin functional groups. Other reactions are dependent on the intra- or intermolecular approach of reactive, functional groups. Thus it can be argued that 'stereopopulation control' [77] and 'effective molarity' [78] are important determinants for protein chemical degradation. The effects of excipients and insulin physical state on the chemical transformation of insulin are probably all governed via an influence on the local conformational structure around the reacting groups. Constraints upon conformation impede deamidation at residue B3, as has also been observed for deamidation of ribonuclease A [41], of calbindin D_{9k} [26], and of serine hydroxymethyltransferase when compared with its 14-mer amino terminal peptide [29]. On the other hand, restriction of the tertiary and quaternary structure can also result, as in the case of the insulin A-chain cleavage, in cooperative catalytic effects by approximation of active functional groups of potential catalysts. Therefore, three-dimensional structures of proteins are, although in a very complex manner, the main determinants for their chemical degradation.

Acknowledgements

The author is grateful for the excellent technical assistance of Lene Grønlund Andersen and wishes to acknowledge R. E. Hubbard and Xiao Bing, University of York, England, and L. Nørskov-Lauritsen, Novo Nordisk A/S Denmark for their help and advice on the molecular modeling. I am also thankful to P. Balschmidt, Novo Nordisk A/S and G. G. Dodson, University of York, England for helpful discussions.

References

1. Brange J., Langkjær L., Havelund S. and Vølund A. (1992) Chemical stability of insulin: 1. Hydrolytic degradation during storage of pharmaceutical preparations. *Pharm. Res. 9*, 715–726
2. Brange J., Havelund S. and Hougaard P. (1992) Chemical stability of insulin: 2. Formation of higher molecular weight transformation products during storage of pharmaceutical insulin preparations. *Pharm. Res. 9*, 727–734
3. Brange J. and Langkjær L. (1992) Chemical stability of insulin: 3. Influence of excipients, formulation, and pH. *Acta Pharm. Nord. 4*, 149–158
4. Brange J., Hallund O. and Sørensen E. (1992) Chemical stability of insulin: 5. Isolation, characterization and identification of insulin transformation products. *Acta Pharm. Nord. 4*, 223–232
5. Miller H. K. and Waelsch H. (1952) Utilization of glutamine and asparagine and their peptides by micro-organisms. *Nature 169*, 30–31
6. Leach S. J. and Lindley H. (1953) The kinetics of hydrolysis of the amide group in proteins and peptides. Part 1. The acid hydrolysis of l-asparagine and l-asparaginylglycine. *Trans. Faraday Soc. 49*, 915–920
7. Leach S. J. and Lindley H. (1953) The kinetics of hydrolysis of the amide group in proteins and peptides. Part 2. Acid hydrolysis of glycyl- and l-leucyl-l-asparagine. *Trans. Faraday Soc. 49*, 921–925
8. Bender M. L. (1957) General acid-base catalysis in the intramolecular hydrolysis of phthalamic acid. *J. Am. Chem. Soc. 79*, 1258–1259
9. Slobin L. I. (1964) The action of carboxypeptidase A on bovine insulin and related model peptides. Ph.D. Dissertation. University of California, Berkeley
10. Carpenter F. H. (1966) Relationship of structure to biological activity of insulin as revealed by degradative studies. *Am. J. Med. 40*, 750–758
11. Bender M. L. and Neveu M. C. (1958) Intramolecular catalysis of hydrolytic reactions. IV. A comparison of intramolecular and intermolecular catalysis. *J. Am. Chem. Soc. 80*, 5388–5391
12. Dahlgren G. and Simmerman N. L. (1965) The effect of ethyl substitution on the kinetics of the hydrolysis of maleamic and phthalamic acid. *J. Phys. Chem. 69*, 3626–3630
13. Higuchi T., Eberson L. and Herd A. K. (1966) The intramolecular facilitated hydrolytic rates of methyl-substituted succinanilic acids. *J. Am. Chem. Soc. 88*, 3805–3808
14. Kirby A. J. and Lancaster P. W. (1972) Structure and efficiency in intramolecular and enzymic catalysis. Catalysis of amide hydrolysis by the carboxy-group of substituted maleamic acids. *J. Chem. Soc. Perkin 2*, 1206–1214
15. Aldersley M. F., Kirby A. J., Lancaster P. W., McDonald R.S. and Smith C. R. (1974) Intramolecular catalysis of amide hydrolysis by the carboxy-group. Rate determining proton transfer from exter-

nal general acids in the hydrolysis of substituted maleamic acids. *J. Chem. Soc. Perkin 2*, 1487–1495

16. Kluger R. and Lam C.-H. (1976) Rate-determining processes in the hydrolysis of maleanilinic acids in acidic solutions. *J. Am. Chem. Soc.* 98, 4154–4158

17. Kluger R. and Lam C.-H. (1978) Carboxylic acid participation in amide hydrolysis. External general base and general acid catalysis in reactions of norbornenylanilic acids. *J. Am. Chem. Soc.* 100, 2191–2197

18. Sundby F. (1962) Separation and characterization of acid-induced insulin transformation products by paper electrophoresis in 7 M urea. *J. Biol. Chem.* 237, 3406–3411

19. Wright H. T. (1991) Sequence and structure determinants of the nonenzymatic deamidation of asparagine and glutamine residues in proteins. *Protein Eng.* 4, 283–294

20. Aswad D. W. (1984) Stoichiometric methylation of porcine adrenocorticotropin by protein carboxyl methyltransferase requires deamidation of asparagine 25. Evidence for methylation at the α-carboxyl group of atypical l-isoaspartyl residues. *J. Biol. Chem.* 259, 10714–10721

21. Bhatt N. P., Patel K. and Borchardt R. T. (1990) Chemical pathways of peptide degradation. I. Deamidation of adrenocorticotropic hormone. *Pharm. Res.* 7, 593–599

22. Di Donato A., Galletti P. and D'Alessio G. (1986) Selective deamidation and enzymatic methylation of seminal ribonuclease. *Biochemistry* 25, 8361–8368

23. Diaugustini R. P., Gibson B. W., Aberth W., Kelly M., Ferrua C. M., Tomooka Y., Brown C. F. and Walker M. (1987) Evidence for isoaspartyl (deamidated) forms of mouse epidermal growth factor. *Anal. Biochem.* 165, 420–429

24. Voorter C. E., Haard-Hoekman W. A. de, Oetelaar P. J. M. van den, Bloemendal H. and Jong W. W. (1988) Spontaneous peptide bond cleavage in aging α-crystallin through a succinimide intermediate. *J. Biol. Chem.* 263, 19020–19023

25. Kossiakoff A. A. (1988) Tertiary structure is a principal determinant to protein deamidation. *Science* 240, 191–194

26. Chazin W. J., Kördel J., Thulin E., Hofmann T., Drakenberg T. and Forsén S. (1989) Identification of an isoaspartyl linkage formed upon deamidation of bovine calbindin D$_{9k}$ and structural characterization by 2D ^{1}H NMR. *Biochemistry* 28, 8646–8653

27. Ota I. M. and Clarke S. (1989) Calcium affects the spontaneous degradation of aspartyl/asparaginyl residues in calmodulin. *Biochemistry* 28, 4020–4027

28. Violand B. N., Schlittler M. R., Toren P. C. and Siegel N. R. (1990) Formation of isoaspartate 99 in bovine and porcine somatropins. *J. Protein Chem.* 9, 109–117

29. Artigues A., Birkett A. and Schirch V. (1990) Evidence for the *in vivo* deamidation and isomerization of an asparaginyl residue in cytosolic serine hydroxymethyltransferase. *J. Biol. Chem.* 265, 4853–4858

30. Robinson A. B. and Rudd C. J. (1974) Deamidation of glutaminyl and asparaginyl residues in peptides and proteins, In *Current Topics in Cellular Regulation*, Vol. 8 (B. L. Horecker and E. R. Stadtman, Eds.), Academic Press, New York, pp. 247–295

31. Geiger T. and Clarke S. (1987) Deamidation, isomerization and racemization at asparaginyl and aspartyl residues in peptides. Succinimide-linked reactions that contribute to protein degradation. *J. Biol. Chem.* 262, 785–794

32. Capasso S., Mazzarella L., Sica F. and Zagari A. (1989) Deamidation via cyclic imide in asparaginyl peptides. *Peptide Research* 2, 195–200

33. Patel K. and Borchardt R. T. (1990) Chemical pathways of peptide degradation. III. Effect of primary sequence on the pathways of deamidation of asparaginyl residues in hexapeptides. *Pharm. Res.* 7, 787–793

34. Tyler-Cross R. and Schirch V. (1991) Effects of amino acid sequence, buffers, and ionic strength on the rate and mechanism of deamidation of asparagine residues in small peptides. *J. Biol. Chem.* 266, 22549–22556

35. Clarke S. (1987) Propensity for spontaneous succinimide formation from aspartyl and asparaginyl residues in cellular proteins. *Int. J. Peptide Protein Res.* 30, 808–821

36. Stephenson R. C. and Clarke S. (1989) Succinimide formation from aspartyl and asparaginyl peptides as a model for the spontaneous degradation of proteins. *J. Biol. Chem.* 264, 6164–6170

37. Lura R. and Schirch V. (1988) Role of peptide conformation in the rate and mechanism of deamidation of asparaginyl residues. *Biochemistry* 27, 7671–7677

38. Baker E. N., Blundell T. L., Cutfield J. F., Cutfield S. M., Dodson E. J., Dodson G. G., Hodgkin D. M. C., Hubbard R. E., Isaacs N. W., Reynolds C. D., Sakabe K., Sakabe N. and Vijayan N. M. (1988) The structure of 2Zn pig insulin crystals at 1.5 Å resolution. *Phil. Trans. R. Soc.* 319, 369–456

39. Derewenda U., Derewenda Z., Dodson E., Dodson G. G., Reynolds C. D., Smith G. D., Sparks C. and Swenson D. (1989) Phenol stabilizes more helix in a new symmetrical zinc insulin hexamer. *Nature* 338, 594–596

40. Ota I. M. and Clarke S. (1989) Enzymatic methylation of l-isoaspartyl residues derived from aspartyl residues in affinitypurified calmodulin. The role of conformational flexibility in spontaneous isoaspartyl formation. *J. Biol. Chem.* 264, 54–60

41. Wearne S. J. and Creighton T. E. (1989) Effect of protein conformation on rate of deamidation: Ribonuclease A. *Proteins: Struct. Funct. Genet.* 5, 8–12

42. Battersby A. R. and Robinson J. C. (1955) Studies on specific chemical fission of peptide links. Part 1. The rearrangement of aspartyl and glutamyl peptides. *J. Biol. Chem.* 246, 259–269

43. Meinwald Y. C., Stimson E. R. and Scheraga H. A. (1986) Deamidation of the asparaginyl-glycyl sequence. *Int. J. Peptide Protein Res.* 28, 79–84

44. McFadden P. N. and Clarke S. (1987) Convertion of isoaspartyl peptides to normal peptides: Implications for the cellular repair of damaged proteins. *Proc. Natl. Soc. Sci., USA* 84, 2595–2599

45. Tsuda T., Uchiyama M., Sato T., Yoshino H., Tsuchiya Y., Ishikawa S., Ohmae M., Watanabe S., and Miyake Y., 1990, Mechanism and kinetics of secretin degradation in aqueous solutions. *J. Pharm. Sci.* 79, 223–227

46. Johnson B. A., Shirokawa J. M., Hancock W. S., Spellman M. W., Basa L. J. and Aswad D. W. (1989) Formation of isoaspartate at two distinct sites during *in vitro* aging of human growth hormone. *J. Biol. Chem.* 264, 14262–14271

47. Wright H. T. and Robinson A. B. (1982) Cryptic amidase-active sites catalyze deamidation in proteins. In *From cyclotrons to cytochromes. Essays in molecular biology and chemistry.* (Kaplan N. O. and Robinson A., Eds.) Acad. Press, New York, London, pp. 727–743

48. Ernst M. L. and Schmir G. L. (1966) Isoimides. A kinetic study of the reactions of nucleophiles with N-phenylphthalisoimide. *J. Am. Chem. Soc.* 88, 5001–5009

49. Sauers C. K., Marikakis C. A. and Lupton M. A. (1973) Synthesis of saturated isoimides. Reactions of N-phenyl-2,2-dimethylsuccinisoimide with aqueous buffer solutions. *J. Am. Chem. Soc.* 95, 6792–6799

50. Barber J. R. and Clarke S. (1985) Demethylation of protein carboxyl methyl esters: A nonenzymatic process in human erythrocytes. *Biochemistry* 24, 4867–4871

51. Bruice T. C. and Pandit U. K. (1960) The effect of geminal substitution ring size and rotamer distribution on the intramolecular nucleophilic catalysis of the hydrolysis of monophenyl esters of dibasic acids and the solvolysis of the intermediate anhydrides. *J. Am. Chem. Soc.* 82, 5858–5865

52. Bernhard S. A., Berger A., Carter J. H., Katchalski E., Sela M. and Shalitin Y. (1962) Co-operative effects of functional groups in peptides. I. Aspartyl-serine derivatives. *J. Am. Chem. Soc.* 84, 2421–2434

53. Shalitin Y. and Bernhard S. A. (1964) Neighboring effects on ester hydrolysis. I. Neighboring hydroxyl groups. *J. Am. Chem. Soc.* 86, 2291–2292

54. Shalitin Y. and Bernhard S. A. (1966) Cooperative effects of functional groups in peptides. II. Elimination reactions in aspartyl-(O-acyl)-serine derivatives. *J. Am. Chem. Soc. 88*, 4711–4721

55. Teshima G., Stults J. T., Ling V. and Canova-Davis E. (1991) Isolation and characterization of a succinimide variant of methionyl human growth hormone. *J. Biol. Chem. 266*, 13544–13547

56. Hangauer D. G., Monzingo A. F. and Matthews B. W. (1984) An interactive computer graphics study of thermolysin-catalyzed peptide cleavage and inhibition by N-carboxymethyl dipeptides. *Biochemistry 23*, 5730–5741

57. Emdin S. O., Dodson G. G., Cutfield J. M. and Cutfield S. M. (1980) Role of zinc in insulin biosynthesis. Some possible zinc-insulin interactions in the pancreatic B-cell. *Diabetologia 19*, 174–182

58. Chawdhury S. A., Dodson E. J., Dodson G. G., Reynolds C. D., Tolley S. P., Blundell T. L., Cleasby A., Pitts J. E., Tickle I. J. and Wood S. P. (1983) The crystal structure of three non-pancreatic human insulins. *Diabetologia 25*, 460–464

59. Vallee B. L. and Auld D. S. (1990) Zinc coordination, function and structure of zinc enzymes and other proteins. *Biochemistry 29*, 5647–5659

60. Helbig H.-J. (1976) Insulindimere aus der B-Komponente von Insulinpräparationen. Rheinisch-Westfälische Technische Hochschule, Aachen, Germany (dissertation)

61. Kirk K. L. and Cohen L. A. (1972) Intramolecular aminolysis of amides. Effects of electronic variations in the attacking and leaving groups. *J. Am. Chem. Soc. 94*, 8142–8147

62. Brange J., Skelbaek-Pedersen B., Langkjaer L., Damgaard U., Ege H., Havelund S., Heding L. G., Jørgensen K. H., Lykkeberg J., Markussen J., Pingel M. and Rasmussen E. (1987) *Galenics of Insulin: The physico-chemical and pharmaceutical aspects of insulin and insulin preparations.* Springer-Verlag, Berlin, Heidelberg, New York, London, Paris, Tokyo

63. Schlichtkrull J. (1958) Insulin crystals. Chemical and biological studies on insulin crystals and insulin zinc suspensions. Thesis, Ejnar Munksgaard Publisher, Copenhagen

64. Caspar D. L. D. and Badger J. (1991) Plasticity of crystalline proteins. *Current Opinion in Structural Biology 1*, 877–882

65. Bentley G., Dodson G. and Lewitova A. (1978) Rhombohedral insulin crystal transformation. *J. Mol. Biol. 126*, 871–875

66. Blundell T., Dodson G., Hodgkin D. and Mercola D. (1972) Insulin: The structure in the crystal and its reflection in chemistry and biology. *Adv. Protein Chem. 26*, 279–402

67. Balschmidt P., Hansen F. B., Dodson E. J., Dodson G. G. and Korber G. (1991) Structure of porcine insulin cocrystallized with clupeine Z. *Acta Cryst. B47*, 975–986

68. Cecil R. and McPhee J. R. (1959) The sulfur chemistry of proteins. *Adv. Protein Chem. 14*, 255–389

69. Florence T. M. (1980) Degradation of protein disulphide bonds in dilute alkali. *Biochem J. 189*, 507–520

70. Helmerhorst E. and Stokes G. B. (1983) Generation of acid-stable and protein-bound persulfide-like residues in alkali- or sulfhydryl-treated insulin by a mechanism consonant with the β-elimination hypothesis of disulfide bond lysis. *Biochemistry 22*, 69–75

71. Cavallini D., Federici G. and Barboni E. (1970) Interaction of protein with sulfide. *Eur. J. Biochem. 14*, 169–174

72. Ryle A. P. and Sanger F. (1955) Disulfide interchange reactions. *Biochem. J. 60*, 535–540

73. Fava A., Iliceto A. and Camera E. (1957) Kinetics of the thiol-disulfide exchange. *J. Am. Chem. Soc. 79*, 833–838

74. Jones A. J., Helmerhorst E. and Stokes G. B. (1983) The formation of dehydroalanine residues in alkali-treated insulin and oxidized glutathione. *Biochem. J. 211*, 499–502

75. Brange J. and Langkjær L. (1993) Insulin structure and stability. In *Stability and Characterization of Protein and Peptide Drugs – Case Histories* (Wang J. and Pearlman R. Eds.) Plenum Publ. Corp., New York. (In press)

76. Di Donato A. and D'Alessio G. (1981) Heterogeneity of bovine seminal ribonuclease. *Biochemistry 20*, 7232–7237

77. Milstien S. and Cohen L. A. (1972) Stereopopulation control. I. Rate enhancement in the lactonizations of o-hydroxyhydrocinnamic acids. *J. Am. Chem. Soc. 94*, 9158–9165

78. Kirby A. J. (1980) Effective molarities for intramolecular reactions. In *Advances in physical organic chemistry. Vol. 17* (Gold V. and Bethell D., Eds) Acad. Press, London, New York, pp. 183–278

79. McKerrow J. H. and Robinson A. B. (1971) Deamidation of asparaginyl residues as a hazard in experimental protein and peptide procedures. *Anal. Biochem. 42*, 565–568

Received May 5, 1992.
Accepted May 18, 1992.

Reproduced from *Acta Pharmaceutica Nordica*, 4(4):223–232,
1992. Copyright Swedish Pharmaceutical Society. With permission.

Chemical stability of insulin

5. Isolation, characterization and identification of insulin transformation products

Jens Brange*, Ole Hallund and Else Sørensen

Novo Research Institute, Novo Alle, DK-2880 Bagsværd, Denmark

During storage of insulin formulated for therapy, minor amounts of various degradation and covalent di- and polymerization products are formed [1–3]. The main chemical transformation products were isolated from aged preparations and characterized chemically and biologically. The most prominent products formed in neutral medium were identified as a mixture of deamidation products hydrolyzed at residue B3, namely isoAsp B3 and Asp B3 derivatives. A hydrolysis product formed only in crystals of insulin zinc suspensions containing a surplus of zinc ions in the supernatant was identified as an A8–A9 cleavage product. The small amounts of covalent insulin dimers (CID) formed in all formulations were shown to be a heterogenous mixture of 5–6 different CIDs with a composition dependent on the pharmaceutical formulation. The chemical characteristics of the CIDs indicate that they are formed through a transamidation reaction mainly between the B-chain N-terminal and one of the four amide side-chains of the A chain. Gln^{A15}, Asn^{A18} and, in particular, Asn^{A21} participate in the formation of such isopeptide links between two insulin molecules. The covalent insulin-protamine products (CIPP) formed during storage of NPH preparations presumably originate from a similar reaction between the protamine N-terminal with an amide in insulin. Covalent polymerization products, mainly formed during storage of amorphously suspended insulin at higher temperature, were shown to be due to disulfide interactions. Biological *in vivo* potencies relative to native insulin were less than 2% for the split-(A8–A9)-product and for the covalent disulfide exchange polymers, 4% for the CIPP, approximately 15% for the CIDs, whereas the B3 derivatives exhibited full potency. Rabbit immunization experiments revealed that none of the insulin transformation products had significantly increased immunogenicity in rabbits.

During the last two decades modern chromatographic processes have been introduced and become standard methods for purification of insulin used for pharmaceutical preparations. This development has led to insulin of very high purity since contaminants are virtually undetectable by the classic methods of size exclusion chromatography and disc electrophoresis; even when analyzed by the sensitive high performance liquid chromatography (HPLC) methods the purity is normally better than 99.5%. Therefore, insulin is today probably the purest protein available and the same is true for the insulin in freshly prepared insulin preparations. However, like other proteins, insulin is not a stable entity but is liable to modification by chemical reactions with molecules in its vicinity. Thus, during storage and use of pharmaceutical preparations, insulin is degraded by hydrolytic reactions or is transformed by formation of intermolecular covalent bonds with other insulin molecules or with auxiliary substances leading to higher molecular weight transformation (HMWT) products.

In four previous papers in this series, studies on chemical transformation of insulin during storage have been reported [1–4]. Four major hydrolysis products are formed in different insulin preparations, as revealed by disc electrophoresis, all appearing anodically to the insulin band on the gel [1]. Band 1 is formed in acid formulations and has been identified as monodesamido-(A21)-insulin [5, 6]. Band 2 only appears during storage of certain insulin zinc suspensions (IZS) containing rhombohedral crystals. Band 3 and 4 are formed in most neutral formulations but in varying amounts. In acid solutions, a fifth band starts to appear after storage for longer time. This band 5 most likely contains didesamido-insulins [5]. Minor amounts of HMWT products are formed in all preparations, mostly in the form of covalent insulin dimers (CID), but in protamine-containing preparations an additional peak eluted in front of the CID peak in size exclusion chromatography. In addition, covalent oligo- and polymerization products can be observed after storage at temperatures above 25°C [2].

The purpose of the present work was to isolate and identify the most prominent of these insulin transformation products, and to characterize them with special emphasis on their biological and immunological properties.

---

* Correspondence

Experimental

Materials

Insulins used for the studies were monocomponent (MC) insulin. Potency: 28 IU/mg (dry weight) corresponding to 1.68×10^8 IU/mol. Zn^{2+} content: 0.4% (w/w of insulin) corresponding to approximately 2 Zn^{2+} per insulin hexamer. Insulin purity: > 99.5% by reversed phase HPLC (RP-HPLC). Distilled water (if necessary degassed by evacuation prior to use) was used for all chromatographic eluents and electrophoretic buffers. Leucine aminopeptidase (type III-CP) was obtained from Sigma and was dialyzed before use (5 mM barbital buffer, 3 mM $MgCl_2$, pH 8) and activated for 30 min at 40°C. Dansylchloride in a purity of >98% was obtained from Fluka AG. All other chemicals were either official (Ph. Eur. or B.P.) or analytical grade. Silica gel plates for TLC were from Merck, Germany. Ampholine pH 5–8 was obtained from LKB, Sweden. Percentages are w/v if not otherwise stated.

Methods

Accelerated ageing of insulin preparations

Insulin preparations in the different formulations were prepared according to the various pharmacopoeias and stored at elevated temperatures. Isolation of insulin (and the insulin derivatives formed during storage) from the pharmaceutical insulin preparations was performed as described earlier [1].

Separation, isolation and purification of insulin derivatives

Initial separation according to molecular weight was performed by size exclusion chromatography (SEC) on Sephadex G-50 (fine or superfine) columns (5×80 or 15×130 cm) in 1 M acetic acid at 20°C. The collected eluent fractions were stored at 4°C. HMWT products were re-chromatographed on Biogel P-30 or P-60 (100–200 mesh) columns (2.5×50 or 5×80 cm) in 1–5 M acetic acid. After dilution to < 0.5 M acetic acid, the individual HMWT products were isolated by lyophilization. The fractions from the SEC columns, containing insulin and the hydrolytic degradation products, were salted out (17% NaCl) at 5–10°C, and after centrifugation the isolated material was immediately re-dissolved in 20 mM HCl, followed by precipitation at pH 6 by addition of zinc acetate to 10 mM Zn^{2+} as described earlier [1]. After centrifugation the isolated material was stored at below –20°C.

Hydrolysis products were separated from insulin by anion exchange chromatography on QAE-Sephadex A-25 in 0.1 M TRIS buffer (60% (v/v) ethanol, 125 mM NaCl, pH 8.4) thermostated at 25°C. Elution rate 6.5 cm/h. Material isolated from SEC was dissolved in water by addition of edetic acid (1 mol per mol of insulin+derivatives) and TRIS base to pH 8.4 followed by ethanol to 60% (v/v). Fractions were collected at 6–8°C. Hydrolytic products were precipitated from the relevant fractions, after diluting to 30% ethanol and adjusting pH to 6.0 with HCl, by addition of zinc acetate to 50 mM Zn^{2+}. The mixture was left overnight at 4°C to allow complete precipitation of hydrolytic products which were then isolated by centrifugation, washed with a small amount of 1 mM zinc acetate, and stored at below –20°C without drying.

The individual hydrolysis products were separated by cation exchange chromatography on SP-Sephadex A-25 column in 20 mM citrate buffer (60% ethanol (v/v), 105 mM NaCl, pH 3.8) thermostated at 20°C. Elution rate 6.5 cm/h. Sometimes, an ionic strength gradient (I = 0.1–0.2) was used after elution of the first hydrolysis products. The mixture of hydrolysis products isolated from the anion chromatography was dissolved in distilled water by addition of citric acid and edetic acid, followed by ethanol to 60% (v/v). Fractions were collected at 6–8°C. After evaporation in vacuum of most of the ethanol from the pooled fractions, hydrolytic products were salted out, followed by redissolution and zinc-precipitation as described above, and after lyophilization stored at below –20°C. Zinc-free products were obtained by desalting on Sephadex G-10 in 1 M acetic acid followed by lyophilization.

In all chromatographic separations eluates were monitored by the absorbance at 280 nm in a 1 cm quartz cuvette.

Analytical characterization

RP-HPLC was performed on Lichrosorp C_{18} columns (4×250 mm) at 40°C. Flow 1 ml/min. Reservoir A: 0.2 M sodium sulfate, 0.04 M phosphoric acid, 0.02 M ethanolamine, acetonitrile 10%. Reservoir B: acetonitrile 50%. Elution: isocratically 30 min with 44% B, followed by gradient (30–70 min) to 66% B. Eluates were monitored by the absorbance at 214 nm.

Electrophoresis on cellulose acetate membranes was performed in Microzone electrophoresis cells using Duostat power supply (Beckman, USA). Buffers were at pH 8.6: 0.05 M barbital buffer (150 V for 1–2 h), at pH 1.9: 15% (v/v) formic acid, 10% (v/v) acetic acid and 4 M urea (150 V for 1–2 h). Staining was performed with 1% amido black in 7% (v/v) acetic acid or, for A-chain S-sulfonates, 5% ethacridine in 0.5 M sodium bicarbonate. For alkaline electrophoresis, edetic acid was added (to 1 mM) to Zn^{2+} containing sample solutions.

N-terminal analysis was performed by the dansyl (DNS) technique as described by Gros and Labouesse [7] with identification of the DNS amino acid derivatives by 2-dimensional TLC, according to Seiler and Wiechmann [8].

Amino acid analysis was performed on a Durrum D-500 analyzer as described by Jacobsen et al. [9].

Polyacrylamide disc gel electrophoresis (PAGE) at pH 8.6 was performed as described earlier [1]. PAGE at pH 4.5 was performed on gel plates according to Reisfeld et al. [10]. The solutions used for preparing the gels and dissolving the samples, were 8 M with respect to urea. The electrophoresis was run for 3 h. The gels were stained for 2–4 h in a 1% solution of amido black in 7% (v/v) acetic acid, and excess dye was removed by washing with 3% (v/v) acetic acid.

Analytical isoelectric focusing in polyacrylamide gel was carried out in 0.5×12 cm glass tubes at 4°C as described by Wrigley [11] with the following modifications: The solutions used for preparing the gels were 8 M with respect to urea and Ampholine pH 5–8 was used. Samples were dissolved in DMSO containing 8% (v/v) of a sucrose solution (25 g sucrose + 16 ml water). The focusing was performed at 4°C with prefocusing for 3.5 hour, and 10–250 µg protein was applied in 50 µl. Fixation of the protein bands was carried out in 15% trichloroacetic acid. Some of the gels were cut into 5 mm disks and placed in 1 ml of distilled water for several hours, followed by measurement of pH.

Identification

Sulfitolysis of insulin derivatives was performed in 130 mM sodium sulfite, 65 mM sodium tetrathionate at pH 9.0 which, according to Cecil and Loening [12], will leave the A-chain internal disulfide bridge intact. After 3 h at 37°C, urea was added to 8 M, and the A- and B-chains were separated on Sephadex G-75 in 50% (v/v) acetic acid according to Varandani [13], or on Sephadex G-50 in 50 mM ammonium carbonate at pH 9.0.

N-terminal sequence

Analyses on the PAGE band 2 compound and its A-chain S-sulfonate derivative, were performed by Edman degradation using an Applied Biosystems model 470A gas-phase sequencer, with quantification of the phenylthiohydantoin amino acids by RP-HPLC on an IBM cyano column in a Hewlett Packard liquid chromatograph model 1084B equipped with a variable UV-detector model 79875, as described by Moody et al. [14].

Analyses on the B-chain S-sulfonate derivatives of the compounds in PAGE bands 3 and 4 were performed by a manual dansyl-Edman degradation technique as described by Gray [15], with identification of the amino acids by TLC as described above under N-terminal analysis.

Leucine aminopeptidase (LAP) degradation was performed on approximately 100 nmol B-chain S-sulfonate (in 0.1 ml 5 mM barbital buffer) with 0.1 mg activated LAP for 16 and 28 h at 40°C [16]. Amino acids were isolated by dialysis followed by evaporation in vacuum, and identified by the DNS technique as described above (porcine insulin derivatives), or by amino acid analysis (bovine insulin derivatives) as described above.

Biological characterization

Biological potency in vivo was estimated either by the mouse blood glucose assay (Ph. Eur. modified by using 32 mice per assay and with blood sampling before and 30, 60 and 90 min after injection) or the mouse convulsion assay after Ph. Eur.

The covalent polymerization products exhibited strongly protracted blood glucose lowering effect. In the bioassay, they were therefore compared with a long-acting protamine-insulin preparation used as the standard.

Immunogenicity studies were performed in groups of 10 rabbits immunized twice weekly with 0.8 mg insulin and insulin split-(A8–A9)-product with Freund's incomplete adjuvant for approximately 3 months, as described earlier [17]. Blood was drawn every 2–3 weeks and insulin antibodies were estimated as the percent bound insulin in sera diluted 1:3.

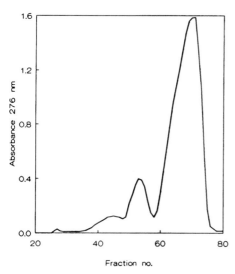

Fig. 1. *Size exclusion chromatography in 1 M acetic acid on 15×130 cm Sephadex G-50 fine, of crystalline IZS (U 40, porcine) aged for one year at 37°C.*
The crystals from 3.6 l preparation (corresponding to 5.4 g insulin plus derivatives) were isolated by centrifugation, dissolved in 150 ml 2.5 M acetic acid and applied on the column. Fractions of 260 ml were collected. Insulin plus hydrolytic degradation products in the main peak were isolated as described in the experimental section and further separated by ion exchange chromatographies (examples in Figs. 2–4). The small peak 1 contains insulin polymers, peak 2 covalent insulin trimers, and peak 3 CID.

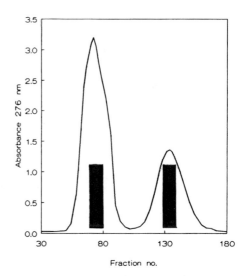

Fig. 2. *Anion exchange chromatography on QAE-Sephadex A-25 (5×30 cm), of insulin plus hydrolytic degradation products formed in neutral regular insulin (containing NaCl and methylparaben) during storage for seven months at 37°C.*
Initial removal of HMWT products was performed by SEC (see Fig. 1). Insulin plus derivatives (3.2 g) were applied in 75 ml buffer and 25 ml fractions were collected. Inserts are the PAGE (pH 8.6) pattern of the two peaks (only the lower one third, anodal part of the gel is shown).

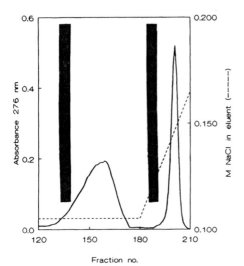

Fig. 3. *Cation exchange chromatography on SP-Sephadex A-25 (2.5×35 cm), of 150 mg of the insulin hydrolytic degradation products isolated from the second peak in Fig. 2.*
The product mixture was applied in 7 ml buffer and 20 ml fractions were collected. Inserts are the PAGE (pH 8.6) pattern of the two peaks. The upper, weak band on the gels is proinsulin used as internal standard (Ref. 1).

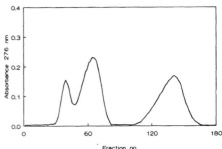

Fig. 4. *Cation exchange chromatography on SP-Sephadex A-25 (2.5×32 cm), with 0.13 M NaCl used in the eluent, of 230 mg of insulin hydrolytic degradation products formed in IZS, mixed (porcine) during storage for one year at 25°C, and previously separated from HMWT products and insulin (see Figs. 1 and 2).*
The mixture was applied in 13 ml buffer and 20 ml fractions were collected. The first and second peak contain PAGE band 4 and 3 products, respectively. The last eluted peak contains the PAGE band 2 product.

Physico-chemical characterization

Hydrolysis products

Electrophoresis at slightly alkaline pH showed the same relative mobility of the different derivatives as in PAGE, except for the product in PAGE band 2 which migrated less towards the anode than insulin. At acid pH, the product in band 2 showed less electrophoretic mobility toward the cathode, band 3 the same mobility, and bands 1, 4 and 5 moved slightly farther than the parent insulin.

Results and discussion

Isolation

Three consecutive runs on different chromatographic columns were necessary in order to obtain the hydrolysis products in pure form. Figs. 1–4 show examples of such runs. The peak on the SP-Sephadex chromatogram corresponding to band 3 on the disc gel always contained smaller amounts of monodesamido-(A21)-insulin (Fig. 3 and 4) which co-eluted with the band 3 compound. As this Asp^{A21} derivative had not been formed in significant amounts during ageing of the neutral preparations, it was most likely formed during the SEC in 1 M acetic acid (Fig. 1).

The HMWT products (Fig. 1) were often re-chromatographed on smaller dimension SEC and RP-HPLC columns. Fig. 5 shows such a re-run on Biogel P-30 of the HMWT products formed in Isophane (NPH) insulin. The HMWT products could be separated into four different peaks and each peak contains several products, as can be observed from the PAGE inserts. The first two peaks contain heterogenous products with an electrophoretic mobility between that of protamine sulfate and CID. Peak 3 contains a mixture of covalent insulin oligomers and protamine sulfate, and peak 4 consists of CIDs.

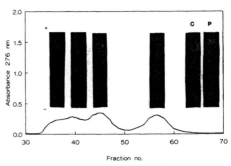

Fig. 5. *Re-chromatography (SEC) in 5 M acetic acid on Biogel P-30 (5×60 cm) of the HMWT products formed in Isophane (NPH) insulin (U 40, porcine) during storage for five years at 25°C.*
The HMWT products (12 mg) were applied in 1 ml, and 2 ml fractions were collected. Inserts are the PAGE (pH 4.5) pattern of the individual peaks + standards (P = protamine, C = CID).

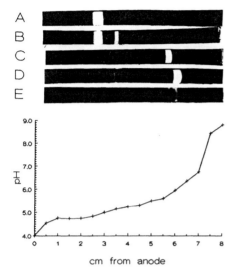

cm from anode

Fig. 6. *Isoelectric focusing of various insulin hydrolytic degradation products.*
A) Peak 1 from Fig. 3 (PAGE band 4); B) Peak 2 from Fig. 3 (PAGE band 3); C) Peak 3 from Fig. 4 (PAGE band 2); D) Insulin (porcine, once crystallized with desamido-insulin-(A21)-insulin as the most prominent impurity); E) Mixture of C and D.
The curve shows the mean of pH measurements on two different gels from the focusing experiment.

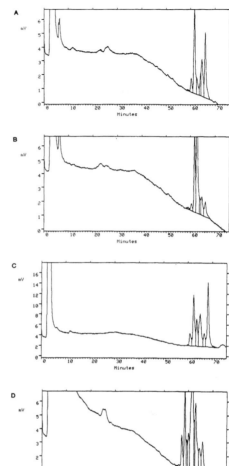

Fig. 7. *Re-chromatography on RP-HPLC of the CID fractions from SEC separations isolated from different, aged porcine insulin preparations (see Fig. 1).*
A) Neutral insulin solution (U 40, formulated with NaCl and methylparaben) stored for 7.5 years at 15°C + 2 months at 37°C.
B) IZS, amorphous (U 40) stored for 7.5 years at 15°C + 2 months at 37°C.
C) IZS, crystalline (U 40) stored for 16 years at 15°C + 2 months at 37°C.
D) Isophane (NPH) insulin (U 40) stored for 12 years at 4°C.

N-terminal and amino acid analyses on the different hydrolysis products showed no differences from the parent species of insulin.

Isoelectric focusing (Fig. 6) revealed that the insulin derivatives in PAGE band 1 had an isoelectric point (IP) approximately 0.4 lower than insulin (IP 5.4), whereas the derivative in band 2 showed an IP quite similar to insulin. However, by isoelectric focusing of a mixture of this derivative and insulin, an 0.05 lower IP of the band 2 compound was demonstrated. The derivatives in PAGE bands 3 and 4 both showed an IP approximately 0.7 lower than insulin.

HMWT products

HMWT formation is only slightly influenced by the species of insulin but varies with the composition and formulation of the preparations [2]. CID peaks from SEC chromatographies of aged samples of different types of preparations were re-chromatographed on RP-HPLC C_{18} columns and, as shown in Fig. 7, the CIDs are heterogenous mixtures of products. Two to five main peaks (> 10% of total) and two to five minor peaks

(≤ 10% of total) can be identified, but the distribution of the individual peaks varies with the type of preparation. Also, the covalent oligo- and polymers formed in amor-

A
B
C
D

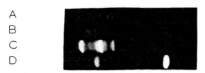

Fig. 8. *Isoelectric focusing of the fractions isolated from SEC on amorphous IZS (U 40, porcine) stored for two months at 37°C.*
A) *Polymers (MW 25–50 kD).*
B) *Oligomers (MW 15–25 kD).*
C) *CID fraction (MW 10–15 kD).*
D) *Insulin plus hydrolysis products.*

phous IZS are highly heterogenous, as revealed by iso-electric focusing (Fig. 8).

Identification

Hydrolysis products

The different hydrolysis products were cleaved into A- and B-chain S-sulfonates by sulfitolysis, and analyses of these derivatives by electrophoresis at pH 8.6 showed that the chemical modifications in the PAGE bands 1 and 2 products were in the A-chain of the products, whereas the B-chain was the location of change in the products contained in bands 3 and 4. The insulin derivative in band 1 has earlier been identified as desamido-(A21)-insulin [5]. Sequence determination by manual Edman degradation on the isolated B-chain S-sulfonates of the two products in bands 3 and 4 clearly showed an Asp-residue in position B3 of the band 3 product as compared to the Asn-residue in the insulin B-chain S-sulfonate. However, only two residues (Phe and Val) were detected in 4 cycles of Edman degradation of the B-chain from the product in band 4. This result indicated an isopeptide bond in B3, which will prevent further degradation by the Edman technique [15]. The existence of an isopeptide bond between B3 and B4 of the product in band 4 from porcine insulin was confirmed by LAP enzymatic hydrolysis. This exopeptidase only cleaves α-peptide bonds [16], and only Phe and Val were released during 28 h treatment of the B-chain from the band 4 product. In contrast, B-chains from insulin and from the band 3 product released several more amino acids during similar LAP treatment, including Asp from the band 3 derivative and Asn from insulin B-chain. Whereas porcine and human insulin during storage in neutral solution form the products in bands 3 and 4 in a ratio of approximately 1:2, bovine insulin appears to form the band 3 product only [1]. Although the cation chromatography has proven the presence of two products (in the same ratio 1:2) in this one band, it was of interest to examine the nature of these products. B-

chains from these products, together with the B-chain from bovine insulin, were therefore treated with LAP as described above. The results of amino acid analyses of the hydrolysates are shown in Table 1. It will appear that amino acids until Tyr B16 have been liberated from the insulin B-chain, which is in good agreement with the 12–13 residues observed by Hill and Smith after 24 hours LAP hydrolysis at 37°C. The B-chain from the band 3, peak 1 product deviated by the appearance of Asp in the hydrolysate, and by lower yields of the amino acids following Asp^{B3} in the sequence, which is consistent with reported lower rate of release of Asp by LAP [16]. However, significant amounts of residues can be observed until residue B16 (Tyr). In sharp contrast, only 2 residues (Phe and Val) are cleaved from the band 3, peak 2 product since only traces of other amino acids were detected. Together these results demonstrate that the band 3 insulin derivative contains an Asp^{B3} residue whereas in the band 4 derivative (or bovine band 3, peak 2 derivative) this residue is transformed into $isoAsp^{B3}$.

N-terminal as well as sequence analyses on the band 2 product from bovine insulin and its A-chain S-sulfonate (isolated on Sephadex G-75) clearly demonstrated that an additional N-terminal (Ser) was present in the A-chain. This offers two possibilities for cleavage of the A-chain, namely between A8 and A9 or between A11 and A12. The results of the sequencing (Table 2) clearly demonstrate that the cleavage has occurred between A8 and A9.

HMWT products

N-terminal analyses on the CID formed in different insulin preparations all showed the same two N-termi-

Table 1. *Amino acid analysis on leucine aminopeptidase (LAP) hydrolyzed B-chains from bovine insulin and PAGE band 3 derivatives of bovine insulin.*

Amino acid	Insulin		Band 3 derivative, SP-Sephadex peak 1		Band 3 derivative, SP-Sephadex peak 2	
	nmol	mol/mol B-chain	nmol	mol/mol B-chain	nmol	mol/mol B-chain
Ala	91	0.7	42	0.3	7	0.05
Arg	9	<0.1	6	<0.1	<1	<0.1
Asp	4	0.03	38	0.3	3	0.02
Glu	100	0.8	46	0.4	11	0.1
Gly	158	1.2	64	0.5	8	<0.1
His	140	1.1	54	0.4	2.6	<0.1
Leu	352	2.7	156	1.2	14	0.1
Lys	9	<0.1	4	<0.1	2.5	<0.1
Phe	132	1.0	126	1.0	130	1.0
Tyr	98	0.8	21	0.2	10	<0.1
Val	280	2.1	203	1.6	150	1.1

LAP hydrolysis of the B-chain S-sulfonates was performed as described in the experimental section and aliquots containing 130 nmol of the hydrolyzed peptides were used for the amino acid analyses.

Table 2. *Sequence analyses.*

A) PAGE band 2 product:

PTH[a] amino acid	1	2	3	4	5	6	7	8 (pmol)	9	10	11	12	13	14	15
								Cyclus number							
Ala				40	31		34	164	101	56	36			257	155
Asn			733	124	1					597	131		184	105	71
Gln				729	870	72	614	84							
Glu		17	7	604	274	43	170	26	274	58	22		173	75	33
Gly	820	27						607	99	31					
His			14	60	320	82				148	80				
Ile		870	113	30											
Leu				5	723	779	161	581	112	41	395	116	123	42	276
Phe	892	28		20					65						
Ser	90			115	28				51						
Tyr						717	79				574	73	51		
Val		1757	963	248	13		46	25	48	27		252	266	75	33

B) A-chain S-sulfonate of PAGE band 2 product:

PTH[a] amino acid	1	2	3	4	5	6	7	8 (pmol)	9	10	11	12	13	14
								Cyclus number						
Asn										90	149	104	28	129
Gln					304	138	96	317	141	18				
Glu				261	141	44	19	85	119	208	37	21		
Gly	435	140	46	28										
Ile		325	120	16										
Leu					143	491	64	120	466	126	19	24		
Ser	192	27		17	78	11								
Tyr					37	154	265	93	40	18	53	386	65	54
Val		957	599	124	16	12								

[a] PTH=phenylthiohydantoin

nals as insulin (Phe and Gly). Sulfitolysis of the CID fraction from SEC chromatography of aged crystalline IZS, (from Fig. 1), followed by size exclusion chromatography on Sephadex G-75 in acetic acid, gave an appa-

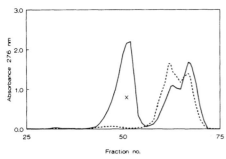

Fig. 9. *SEC on Sephadex G-50 (2.5×40 cm) at pH 9 of sulfitolyzed CID (60 mg) isolated from aged crystalline IZS ——, and sulfitolyzed insulin (40 mg) - - - - -. Fractions of 2 ml were collected.*

The first peak (Peak X) contains a mixture of A–A and A–B chain S-sulfonates in a ratio of 1:2 (Table 3) linked through non-disulfide bonds. Peaks 2 and 3 contain A- and B-chain S-sulfonates, respectively.

rent 50% reduced yield of the A-chain as compared to the B-chain. When, instead, the sulfitolyzed products were separated on Sephadex G-50 at pH 9, 50% of the applied material eluted in an additional peak (peak X) in front of the A- and B-chains (Fig. 9) and a reduced yield of the A-chain was still observed. N-terminal analysis on peak X showed the same two N-terminals as intact insulin but with a tendency towards reduced amounts of Phe. Electrophoresis at pH 1.9 revealed that two main components in peak X had an electrophoretic mobility approximately midway between the A- and B-chain S-sulfonates whereas a minor component (approximately 30% of the total) moved ahead of the A-chain. Electrophoresis at pH 8.6 showed essentially the same pattern, but the intermediate moving components were divided into two major and one minor components. Essentially the same electrophoresis pattern applied to the CID fraction isolated from aged amorphous IZS. Amino acid analysis on peak X from amorphous as well as crystalline IZS showed a composition closely corresponding to one B-chain of insulin plus two A-chains of insulin (Table 3). On the basis of these results, together with reports on the composition of covalent insulin dimers isolated from crude insulin [18], it is reasonable to suggest that the covalent dimers for-

Table 3. Amino acid analysis of peak X (Fig. 9) from SEC on sulfitolyzed covalent insulin dimer isolated from different, aged porcine insulin preparations.

Amino acid	Peak X derived from:		Theory:
	IZS, crystalline	IZS, amorphous	1 B-chain+ 2 A-chains
Ala	2.10	2.10	2
Arg	1.04	1.04	1
Asx	5.25	5.41	5
Cys½	8.51	8.59	10
Glx	11.4	11.5	11
Gly	5.21	5.24	5
His	2.01	2.04	2
Ile	2.44	2.61	4
Leu	8.35	8.66	8
Lys	0.92	0.87	1
Phe	2.98	2.97	3
Pro	1.02	1.08	1
Ser	4.92	5.09	5
Thr	3.02	3.15	3
Tyr	5.95	6.13	6
Val	4.29	4.35	5

The figures are the ratios calculated on basis of Lys=Arg=Pro=1.

med during storage of neutral insulin preparations are partly (2/3) formed by a reaction of the N-terminal B-chain with side-chain amido groups in the A-chain of another insulin molecule (A–B dimer), and partly (1/3) by a reaction of the A-chain N-terminal from one molecule with similar amido groups in another A-chain (A-A dimer). Computer graphic studies have shown that the most likely reacting amido groups are Gln^{A15}, Asn^{A18} and Asn^{A21} [4]. The marked heterogeneity of the CID fraction mentioned earlier, together with the fact that the CID formation is halved when the A21 amido group is deamidated and hence unlikely to react [4], suggests that A21 is the main reacting group. The other half

of the CID fraction probably consists of products linked (A-B and A-A) through A15 and A18. This gives six theoretical possibilities for CID products which is consistent with the number of observed peaks in the RP-HPLC chromatogram (Fig. 7).

Re-chromatography of the CIPP peak from an aged Isophane (NPH) preparation by RP-HPLC revealed at least six poorly separated peaks. The results of amino acid analysis on the CIPP peak demonstrated that its composition closely corresponded to one insulin molecule + one protamine molecule. The main link between them probably originates from aminolysis reactions (transamidation) by the N-terminal amino group of protamine with amides in the insulin molecule as described for CID formation [4].

Biological properties

In vivo potency

The biological potencies of the different hydrolytic decomposition and HMWT products are shown in Table 4. The deamidation products all have full or nearly full in vivo potency. Thus, the potency of a 2:1 mixture of the $isoAsp^{B3}$ and Asp^{B3} derivatives is not significantly different from the parent molecule, which is consistent with the fact that 2–3 residues can be removed from the B-chain N-terminal without loss of potency [19]. Desamido-(A21)-insulin, however, shows a tendency to reduced potency but only that of the bovine variety reaches statistical significance. This result agrees with earlier reports [20, 21] although a somewhat lower potency (60%) for bovine desamido-(A21)-insulin has been reported [22]. The reduced potency is probably related to conformational changes leading to exposure of hydrophobic residues, as indicated by the stronger

Table 4. Biological in vivo potency of transformation products formed in different insulin preparations.

Product[a]	Preparation[b]	Insulin species	Bioassay[c] method	Potency[d] IU/mg (95% conf. lim.)	Potency relative to insulin
MDI-(A21)	Acid solution	porcine	MCA+ MBGA	24.4 (23.5–25.4)	92%
		bovine		22.5 (21.4–23.4)	85%
MDI-(B3)[e]	Neutral Regular	porcine	MCA	25.9 (22.6–30.0)	97%
Split-(A8–A9)	IZS, crystalline	bovine	MBGA	0.58 (0.37–0.77)	2%
CID	IZS, crystalline	porcine	MBGA	4.4 (3.5–5.4)	15%
CIPP	Isophane (NPH)	bovine	MBGA	1.2 (0.9–1.5)	4%
Polymer[f]	IZS, amorphous	porcine	MBGA	0.4 (0.2–0.6)	1.5%

[a]) MDI=Monodesamido-insulin; CID=Covalent insulin dimer; CIPP=Covalent insulin-protamine product. [b] IZS=Insulin zinc suspension; NPH=Neutral protamine Hagedorn. [c] MCA=Mouse convulsion assay; MBGA=Mouse blood glucose assay. [d] Based on an insulin derivative containing 14.5% nitrogen. [e] The B3 deamidated product contained 1 part Asp^{B3} and 2 parts $isoAsp^{B3}$ derivative. [f] MW approximately 30 kD.

126

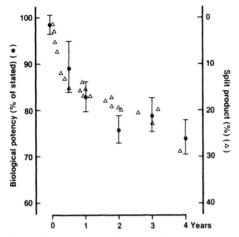

Fig. 10. Biological potency (mouse convulsion assay, mean with 95% confidence intervals) versus content of split – (A8–A9) – product (estimated as described in Ref. 1) during storage at 25°C of crystalline IZS (bovine).

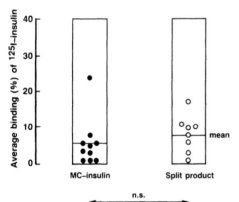

Fig. 11. Groups of rabbits immunized as described in the experimental section. Average binding (area under the curve divided by the number of days of immunization) is plotted for each rabbit.

binding of this derivative relative to that of insulin in RP-HPLC [1].

The split-(A8–A9)-product has very low but significant *in vivo* potency, and, as illustrated in Fig. 10, its formation is the main reason for the decline in biological potency during storage of crystalline IZS. The chain cleavage conceivably may cause considerable perturbation of normal secondary and tertiary structures and exposure of some of the hydrophobic core to the surface of the molecule, as actually indicated by the much larger

retention on the HPLC column [1]. It is interesting to note that the potency, as estimated in an insulin radio-immunoassay (IRI), was as high as 80% relative to insulin. This result confirms that IRI estimates do not give reliable indications of the biological potency of insulin derivatives [23].

The HMWT products all exhibit substantially reduced *in vivo* potency. As larger changes in the N-terminal of the A-chain, in contrast to similar changes in the B-chain, normally lead to a substantial reduction in potency (19), it is conceivable that, in the heterogenous mixture of CIDs, the A-A-dimer has lower and the A-B-dimer higher potency that the result obtained for the mixture.

Immunological properties

Immunogenicity studies on desamido-(A21)-insulin, CIDs and oligo- and polymers (24), and on desamido-(B3)-insulins and CIPP [25] have shown that these insulin transformation products are not significantly more immunogenic in the animal experiments than the native insulin. Similar studies on the split-(A8-A9)-product are shown in Fig. 11. A tendency towards increased average binding in the group immunized with the split product can be observed but the difference is not statistically significant.

Acknowledgements

The authors wish to acknowledge the skilful technical assistance of Lene Grønlund Andersen, Lene Bramsen, Jessie Frederiksen, Eva Bøg Kristensen, Harriet Markussen and Ebba Ravn. We thank Jørgen Elnegård for the large scale SEC separations, Svend Havelund for the RP-HPLC, Henning Jacobsen for the amino acid analyses, and Lars Thim for the sequence analyses.

References

1. Brange J., Langkjær L., Havelund S. and Vølund A. (1992) Chemical stability of insulin: 1. Hydrolytic degradation during storage of pharmaceutical preparations. *Pharm. Res. 9*, 715–726
2. Brange J., Havelund S. and Hougaard P. (1992) Chemical stability of insulin: 2. Formation of higher molecular weight transformation products during storage of pharmaceutical insulin preparations. *Pharm. Res. 9*, 727–734
3. Brange J. and Langkjær L. (1992) Chemical stability of insulin: 3. Influence of excipients, formulation, and pH. *Acta Pharm. Nord.4*, 149–158
4. Brange J. (1992) Chemical stability of insulin: 4. Kinetics and mechanisms of the chemical transformation in pharmaceutical formulation. *Acta Pharm. Nord. 4*, 209–222
5. Sundby F. (1962) Separation and characterization of acid-induced insulin transformation products by paper electrophoresis in 7 M urea. *J. Biol. Chem. 237*, 3406–3411
6. Slobin L. I. and Carpenter F. H. (1963) The labile amide in insulin: Preparation of desalanine-desamido-insulin. *Biochemistry 2*, 22–28
7. Gros C. and Labouesse. (1969) Study of the dansylation reaction of amino acids, peptides and proteins. *European J. Biochem. 7*, 463–470
8. Seiler N. and Wiechmann J. (1964) Zum Nachweis von Aminosäuren im 10⁻¹⁰-Mol-Masstab. Trennung von 1-Dimethylaminonaphthalin-5-sulfonyl-aminosäuren auf Dünnschicht-chromatogrammen. *Experientia XX/10*, 559–560

9. Jacobsen H., Demandt A., Moody A. J. and Sundby F. (1977) Sequence analysis of porcine gut GLI-1. *Biochim. Biophys. Acta* *493*, 452–459

10. Reisfeld R. A., Lewis U. J. and Williams D. E. (1962) Disc electrophoresis of basic proteins and peptides on polyacrylamide gels. *Nature 195*, 281–283

11. Wrigley C. (1968) Gel electrofocusing – a technique for analyzing multiple protein samples by isoelectric focusing. *Science Tools 15*, 17–23

12. Cecil R. and Loening U. E. (1960) The reactions of the disulphide groups of insulin with sodium sulphite. *Biochem. J. 76*, 146–155

13. Varandani P. T. (1966) A convenient preparation of reduced and S-sulfonated A and B chains of insulin. *Biochim. Biophys. Acta 127*, 246–249

14. Moody A. J., Thim L. and Valverde I. (1984) The isolation and sequencing of human gastric inhibitory peptide (GIP). *FEBS Lett. 172*, 142–148

15. Gray W. R. (1972) Sequence analysis with dansyl chloride. *Methods Enzymol. 25*, 333–344

16. Light A. (1972) Leucine aminopeptidase in sequence determination of peptides. *Methods Enzymol. 25*, 253–262

17. Schlichtkrull J., Brange J., Christiansen A. H., Hallund O., Heding L. G., Jørgensen K. H., Rasmussen S. M., Sørensen E. and Vølund A. (1974) Monocomponent insulin and its clinical implications. *Horm. Metab. Res. (Suppl. Ser.) 5*, 134–143

18. Helbig H.-J. (1976) Insulindimere aus der B-Komponente von Insulinpräparationen. Rheinisch-Westfälische Technische Hochschule, Aachen, Germany (dissertation)

19. Blundell T., Dodson G., Hodgkin D. and Mercola D. (1972) Insulin: The structure in the crystal and its reflection in chemistry and biology. *Adv. Protein Chem. 26*, 279–402

20. Carpenter F. H. (1966) Relationship of structure to biological activity of insulin as revealed by degradative studies. *Am. J. Med. 40*, 750–758

21. Chance R. E. (1972) Amino acid sequences of proinsulins and intermediates. *Diabetes 21* (Suppl. 2), 461–467

22. Easter B. R. D., Sutton D. A. and Drewes S. E. (1978) Crystalline [A21-desamido] bovine insulin. *Hoppe-Seyler's Z. Physiol. Chem. 359*, 1229–1236

23. Pingel M. and Vølund A. (1972) Stability of insulin preparations. *Diabetes 21*, 805–813

24. Schlichtkrull J., Pingel M., Heding L. G., Brange J. and Jørgensen K. H. (1975) Insulin preparations with prolonged effect, In: *Handbook of Experimental Pharmacology, New Series*, Volume XXXII/2 (A. Hasselblatt and F. von Bruchhausen, Eds.) Springer-Verlag, Berlin, Heidelberg, New York, pp. 729–777

25. Brange J., Skelbaek-Pedersen B., Langkjaer L., Damgaard U., Ege H., Havelund S., Heding L. G., Jørgensen K. H., Lykkeberg J., Markussen J., Pingel M. and Rasmussen E. (1987) *Galenics of Insulin: The physico-chemical and pharmaceutical aspects of insulin and insulin preparations.* Springer-Verlag, Berlin, Heidelberg, New York, London, Paris, Tokyo

Received May 13, 1992.
Accepted June 9, 1992.

Lightning Source UK Ltd.
Milton Keynes UK
19 February 2010

150359UK00004B/13/A